CRACKING THE BIKIN

6 Secrets to Permanent

© 2014 KYRIN DUNSTON, MD

Limit of Liability / Disclaimer of Warranty:
While the author and publisher have used their bestir efforts in preparing this book, no representations or warranties are made regarding the accuracy or completeness of the contents of this book. The publisher and author specifically disclaim any implied warranties of fitness for a particular purpose, and make no guarantees whatsoever that you will achieve any particular result. Any case studies that are presented heron do not necessary represent what you should expect to achieve, since weight loss success depends on a variety of factors. The case studies used in this book are composites of actual patient experiences. The names have been changed and the case studies may combine the experiences of more than one patient.

The information presented in this book is in no way intended to replace medical advice, counseling or supervision. Nutrition and fitness must be tailored to the personal needs of each individual with consideration of their personal physical condition and circumstances. The content of this book is not intended as a replacement or substitute for healthcare services a reader may need; is for educational purposes only; and is not intended to treat, diagnose, cure or prevent any disease. The advice and programs in this book may not even be suitable for your situation, and you should consult your own physician as appropriate before starting this or any weight loss program. Nutrition and fitness must be considered in the context of a reader's personal health and in consultation with their primary health care provider. The Bikini Code is a very low calorie diet which should only be undertaken in consultation with your personal physician in consideration of your personal needs, physical condition and health. The information in this book is intended to be used under the guidance and care of a physician. Please consult with your physician prior to starting this or any weight loss program.

Published in Savannah, Georgia by Global Transformational Health Solutions, PC.

ISBN 978-1503103191

Library of Congress Control Number:
(obtaining shortly)

Cover design by:
Ben Marshall
Island 82 Media
ben@ben-marshall.com

Cover photography by:
Josh Brandstetter Jabberpics
jabberpics2@gmail.com

Interior design by:
Scott Fuller
scottfullergd@charter.net

To Robyn —

I dedicate this book to my loving mother
and the original Granola Girl, Jeri Jackson,
who tried to teach me the truth the first time
around and who never said, "I told you so."

*Hope you health
flourish in 2017!*

CONTENTS

Foreword

I MET DR. KYRIN DUNSTON AT A CONFERENCE I WAS GIVING this spring. She is an Obstetrician Gynecologist by training and a passionate wellness expert. In addition, she is a stunning woman. What I didn't know was her story.

When she graciously asked me to read her book, *Cracking the Bikini Code,* I was happy to do it. The title certainly is intriguing and, as a woman, I too am vain and believe that regardless of age, we all want to look and feel our best.

Dr. Dunston's story is not very different from those of the patients I have been seeing over the past 25 years. The difference is that she is a physician and has spent decades learning the science, integrating the pieces and finding solutions. Then, she applied all her knowledge to herself and was so thoughtful and organized that she was able to do the hardest thing anyone of us can do; she explained it so that we can all apply it in our individual lives. To see it as a simple process that involves just the burning desire to wear a Marilyn Monroe white bikini, Dr. Dunston has succeeded in taking us off the couch, away from the oversize clothes and into the world of health, wellness and dis- ease prevention without us even noticing what she was doing.

The book is a gem of information, passion and constant support. The explanations of physiologic and medical information are succinct and clear. They don't make a reader feel overwhelmed. The stepwise fashion in which she peels the onion of health and removes each layer of disease and potential harm to our bodies and mind is wise and well throughout. The book is worth reading and following.

I have no doubt that any woman who still hasn't given up on herself, and I believe none of us ever should, will greatly benefit from this book and remember how a doctor struggled herself to find the answer in wellness. And when she did, she shared it with us and wore a bikini, too.

Thank you, Dr. Dunston.

Erika Schwartz, MD, Founding Director
Better Health Initiative
www.bhionline.org
New York, NY, May, 2014.

Introduction

"It's never too late to wear your first bikini."

— Dr. Kyrin Dunston, physician, proud bikini owner

HELLO, MY NAME IS DR. KYRIN DUNSTON, AND YES, THAT'S me in a bikini at 49 years old, baring it all on the cover of this book. I decided to do this not for vanity's sake, but rather because I wanted to take back the power of the bikini, the most-feared piece of clothing known to womankind.

Why did I fear a few little pieces of fabric? I feared it because, like so many other women in this country, I spent the majority of my life struggling with my weight and health. Topping out at 243 pounds, my former self would have suffered a panic attack at the mere thought of wearing anything more revealing than a muumuu, much less a bathing suit, and certainly never a bikini.

But just a few short years ago, one single day changed my entire life. That day was the day I discovered functional medicine, a revolutionary, all natural approach to health and weight management. Throughout this book, you will learn all about functional medicine (sometimes called restorative, metabolic or anti-aging medicine) and how it can help you achieve all your weight loss goals, while also giving you abundant vitality, energy and health along the way.

But first, I would like to share my story of how functional medicine changed my body, my health, my career and my feelings about modern medicine and health care as a whole. Most importantly, I'd also like to share how it allowed me to Crack the Bikini Code for all the other frustrated, bathing-suit-fearing women out there

I was born and raised in Manhattan and lived with my mother and sister in a pre-war apartment. My mother was not a trained physician, but she had a strong passion for medicine, especially alternative medicine, and health was always a topic in our house.

Growing up, my sister and I used to laugh and call her the Granola Girl because she was always making trips to specialty stores for herbal remedies or scouring the city for fresh vegetables. She paid close attention to her diet, rarely used pharmaceutical drugs and championed the healing properties of minerals and vitamins. Naturally, she was excited when I expressed an interest in medicine at an early age.

With her encouragement, I attended Jefferson Medical School in Philadelphia, where I fell head over heels in love with medicine. I was fascinated with the intricacies of the human body, the latest technologies and disease diagnosis skills. I also loved knowing I would spend my life helping people. I quickly became completely enamored with what I was doing and learning.

During medical school I also got married and had two children. This was not exactly easy as I headed into OB/GYN residency at the Medical Center of Delaware. Residency was demanding to say the least and required many sleepless nights and time away from my family. But my passion for medicine kept me going.

Shortly after completing my residency in 1996, I moved south and opened up my own gynecological practice in Savannah, Georgia. I worked hard, and the practice quickly became successful. Within a short period of time, I had four doctors, 30 employees, a 9,100-square-foot building and multi-million dollar annual revenue.

From the outside, it looked like I was successful and happy, like I was living the American dream. But it was during this time that I noticed my own health start to decline. Somewhere in between opening the practice, having a family and praying for a few hours of sleep, I got fat. As I said, at my biggest I weighed 243 pounds. I used the long hours as an excuse to never exercise and to eat whatever I wanted, whenever I wanted.

But it wasn't just the weight. Symptoms of all kinds were surfacing. I started to feel an intense, constant fatigue that quickly became unbearable. I also began experiencing terrible body aches and pains on a regular basis. My hair started thinning and turned gray, and my nails became brittle.

My lack of energy eventually got so bad that my life consisted solely of eating, sleeping and going to work. My poor kids didn't really have a mother because when I got home from work I would beeline into my pajamas and into my bed. My body was slowly shutting down. After a few years like this, it started to be a real struggle just to make it through the day.

In an effort to help myself, I ran all the typical tests on myself and went to see my doctor. We both agreed that I had borderline high blood pressure, but other than that all my tests were normal according to mainstream medicine standards. While this was an accurate description of one of the symptoms I was experiencing, it didn't explain why I was sick. A cardiologist wanted to put me on medicine, but I refused. I knew in my gut there was more to the story. I knew I was really sick and needed more than just a high blood pressure drug to fix it.

During this time, my emotions also started to go on a roller coaster. I became extremely frustrated with my weight and health and had frequent outbursts due to my inability to fix it using the medicine I had been taught to practice in medical school. I started to lash out at my family and spend time depressed, alone in bed with my two best friends: food and TV. I was still going to work every day, but I was beginning to feel different about medicine. Why wasn't it helping me? Why wasn't it answering my questions?

That is when I really started questioning the type of medicine I was practicing. One day I asked a colleague: Do we really help anybody? I feel like we don't really help. We put people on birth control pills. If that doesn't work, we try another one. If that doesn't work, we do surgery. Then we take one ovary out. If that doesn't work, then we do a hysterectomy. If that doesn't work, we try hormone replacement therapy. Patients are depressed, we put them on anti-depressants, but do we ever find out why they are depressed? No. You're overweight? Do we fix that? No.

My colleague replied that we did help people; that we took away their pain and gave them a better quality of life. I wasn't satisfied.

When things were at their worst, my husband became a full-time caretaker to a depressed woman who couldn't do anything for herself. It was as if he was my parent. I was so dysfunctional I couldn't manage my emotions at all. I couldn't handle life anymore. Quite often, he would have to patch me up before I left the house. He would say, "You can do this. You're going to be okay." At night, he would give me pep talks, cookies, wine or whatever else he thought it would take so I would feel good enough to get up again the next day.

As for self-confidence and worth, I had neither. All I wore were muumuu dresses. I had a big pink one, a big black one and a big flowered one. I wouldn't buy clothes because I wouldn't go shopping, so I wore the same things over and over again. Mostly I wore scrubs. I was in the XXL scrubs by then. In addition, for years on end, my sex life was nonexistent. It was the farthest thing from my mind. I didn't even think about it. No fantasies, nothing. I had no real friends or a social life. In fact, I barely had a life at all. All of this got so bad, I started thinking, If this is what life is, then I'm not sure I want to be living.

Then one day I received a gift from a patient that literally saved my life. It was a book about functional medicine called Breakthrough, written by Suzanne Somers. At first, I couldn't imagine what Chrissy from Three's Company could teach me—a board certified doctor—about medicine. But after keeping it on my nightstand for a few months, I eventually gave it a chance.

The book consisted of interviews with dozens of preeminent scientists and doctors in the field of restorative and functional medicine. They were discussing how you can heal many of your health problems (including weight) using natural remedies rather than chemical drugs. It detailed how the chemicals in pharmaceuticals can actually cause damage to your body, while doing very little to actually heal the problem. Sommers and the doctors gave case after case of how patients could transform their lives, bodies and health in miraculous ways.

They went on to explain that what also makes this practice so different from modern medicine is that the physicians use revolutionary, scientifically advanced tests to check for how your individual cells, the most basic building blocks of your body, are functioning (or not functioning). The tests look at things like ATP (energy) production, hormone regulation, nutrient absorption and other basic, vital functions of health that mainstream doctors are taught in medical school but then promptly told to forget in residency and just prescribe the pill of the day.

I read the book like a mystery novel, unable to put it down. After working in medicine for decades, I knew immediately that what Sommers and the doctors were saying was the absolute truth. I believe we all have a built-in truth meter, and while I knew nothing of functional medicine at the time, I knew what I had read was true. It made me think about the things my mother had been trying to teach me years ago.

After I was done with the book, my very first thoughts were, Oh my God. There actually might be hope for me. I do not have to live this miserable life. It was like a door had been cracked open and a little bit of air and light had come in. For the first time in years, I felt hope for the possibility of a better life. Right then and there I made a decision to find out the truth about my health. I was going to fix whatever was ailing me, no matter what it took. It was the ultimate defining moment.

Desperate for relief, I began performing the functional medicine tests on myself, and I immediately started to get real answers. I discovered I had food intolerances (which everyone has based on their unique genetics and lifestyle) that had been destroying my gastrointestinal tract for decades. I learned how my hormones (which control nearly every vital bodily function) were chronically imbalanced due to the large amount of stress in my life. The tests also showed I had severe yeast overgrowth in my gut, heavy metal toxicity issues and low thyroid function, all of which are extremely common in modern Americans. For the first time, I understood why my body and mind weren't functioning normally on a cellular level.

I kept doing the tests. I also started going to functional medicine conferences around the country where I learned how to treat my ailments naturally, and I started to lose weight and feel better. Then I lost some more weight. Eventually, I got down to 140 pounds, which is less than I weighed in high school. But more than that, I shed most of my symptoms, including fatigue, chronic pain, irritable bowel syndrome, hair loss and depression. And that's because this type of medicine is integrative, meaning it addresses all of your major biological systems together to create lasting, true health. It heals the whole body from the inside out.

As I started shrinking, my patients wanted to know what I was doing, and of course I wanted to share it with them. That's when I started to have another real problem. I would see a 28-year-old girl with polycystic ovarian syndrome (her periods were erratic and painful, she was overweight and had acne) and the modern gynecologist answer is: "Here are some birth control pills. Take these and come back in three months and see me." But then I would feel obligated to say, "But there is another, safer way." Of course they would want to know. So I would get into the conversation about functional medicine.

So many patients became interested in the functional medicine testing that I started offering a few of these tests at my practice. Immediately, my patients started getting results similar to mine. And soon we all wanted to know more, dig deeper and feel even better. But there was no one in the area doing this kind of medicine, and I realized unless I started doing it, no one was going to have a functional medicine practitioner to go see—including me.

Within a short time I started to practice both types of medicine in my mainstream practice. However, because functional medicine appointments require an hour of my time, and traditional appointments take ten minutes, chaos quickly ensued. I designated Wednesday and Friday for functional medicine patients and Monday, Tuesday and

Thursday for mainstream patients. I completely separated the two so there would be no interruptions and patients could choose.

My gynecology practice started weighing heavily on me though. I didn't want to give anyone toxic, synthetic-hormone-laden birth control pills, even if that was what they wanted. I was totally out of integrity. I literally felt like I was being pulled in two. I knew I had to let go of my gynecology practice. It was holding me back, and it was holding back the health of my patients. At first, I was going to try and sell it, but that would take too long, and I couldn't bear the thought of practicing mainstream medicine for even one more day.

Although I was terrified, I closed my GYN practice. I thought, What if I fail? What if I can't sustain myself with this new, out-of-the-box type of medicine? But I felt a higher calling. I knew what was right, and I had to go through with it. I don't have any regrets about it. It was one of the best decisions of my life.

After the final decision was made, I completely committed my life and career to understanding everything there is to know about functional medicine and reeducating myself. I became a member of the Life Extension Foundation (LEF), an organization comprised of preeminent scientists, doctors and other pioneers of functional medicine, and attended many LEF conferences. I also joined the American Academy of Anti-Aging Medicine fellowship program, the Institute of Functional Medicine and the American College for Advancement in Medicine. I studied under other trailblazers such as Eric Braverman, Eldred Taylor, Pamela Smith, Russell Blaylock and David Brownstein.

As I continued learning, my health kept improving. Of course I had times when I caved to certain pressures. I can recall once fixating on and eventually eating a piece of pink birthday cake at a friend's birthday, but I was quickly reminded (mostly by the ensuing stomach cramps) that these things are terrible for your body. And so I let the way I feel dictate the way I live. It is no longer about numbers on a scale; it is about feeling great. That is my number-one motivator. I will never go back to being the sick and depressed woman of my past.

Since fully dedicating myself to my functional medicine practice, True Balance MD, I have seen hundreds of patients lose weight, gain vitality and live an optimally healthy life as well. And after seeing so many patients transform their lives with this medicine, I knew it was my calling to share all I had discovered with others.

That's when I developed the Cracking the Bikini Code program. Throughout the book, you will learn all about the program and the scientific principles behind it. But in short, it is a total health and weight loss system I designed using key principles of functional medicine, inspiration from my personal journey and my wealth of experience in medicine. The secrets in this program are guaranteed to unlock a dynamic, all natural approach to health that is not only guaranteed to make you shed as much weight as you want, but also drastically transform your overall life in the process.

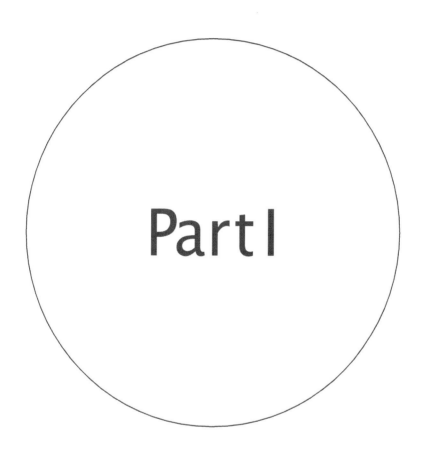

Part I

CHAPTER 1
Be Honest About Your Health

"A girl in a bikini is like having a loaded pistol on your coffee table—there's nothing wrong with it, but it's hard to stop thinking about it."

— Garrison Keillor, author, radio personality

IMAGINE YOU ARE ON A PLANE HEADED TOWARD AN EXOTIC beach vacation (destination of your choosing). When you arrive at the airport, you get off the plane, grab your suitcase and stretch your legs from the long trip while waiting for a taxi to take you to the hotel. While stretching, however, you realize you feel very different than before the flight. You look down, and the first thing you notice is your body—it is much slimmer and more muscular. Perplexed, you scratch your head only to find that your hair is thicker and the skin on your face is softer. As you continue to move, you notice you feel limber and full of energy.

Happy, although a little confused, you get into a taxi and drive across a serene landscape toward your hotel. Looking out of the window, you observe the people, buildings and trees in this new, beautiful place. You crack open the window and smell the salty air, flowers and fresh local foods. The drive is peaceful, and as you make your way, you feel completely relaxed. Your entire body is free from pain. Your mind is also clear and alert.

When you get to the hotel, you reach into your wallet to tip the driver and are startled to find that you have more money than when you boarded the plane. In fact, you have much, much more money. You double-check your driver's license just in case, and yep, it's yours. The hotel bellhop greets you at the car, "Hello, beautiful. We are so pleased and honored to have you stay with us. We have great respect for you and your work." You find it odd that he knows about your work, but you are flattered.

Then he takes you to your room, their largest, most luxurious room on the property. You tip the bellhop generously, because now you can, and open the door to the suite. Inside, a group of loved ones surprise you with a small party and shower you with love. You sit with them and talk and laugh all evening. Then at night you get into your bed, maybe make love with your partner, and drift sweetly off to sleep. You sleep soundly throughout the whole night. When you open your eyes you expect for the whole thing to have been a dream, but it's not. You feel even more vibrant, joyful, healthy and rested than the day before.

Ready to spend a day at the beach with your family and friends, you open your suitcase to get your bathing suit, but all that's there is a bikini. You aren't sure how it got in your suitcase, but everything is going so well you put it on and head to the mirror. You are astonished by what you see. Not only do you look beautiful in the bikini, but you also notice a healthy glow radiating from your entire being. You feel really good in your own skin.

Be honest; wouldn't you love a life like this?

CRACKING THE CODE TO YOUR DREAM LIFE

As you will learn, I am a big fan of visualization techniques, and the one you just read is designed to help you see a detailed picture of the kind of life that you deserve to live, one filled with vitality, love and health (bikini body included). It is the kind of life and health that this book and the entire Bikini Code program is designed to help you get.

Chances are you'd take a flight to that dream life in a heartbeat if given the opportunity. Who wouldn't want the chance to lose weight, shed pain and disease, feel younger, sleep better, have healthier personal relationships and be creative?

In reality, there isn't an airline that I know of offering direct flights to a life like that. But, it doesn't mean there isn't a proven path. In fact, I know of a guaranteed way; I have taken it myself and led hundreds of my patients down it with great success.

That path begins with a three-phase lifestyle plan I created called the Bikini Code program. It's a one-of-a-kind, dynamic approach to weight loss that is guaranteed to naturally help you shed as much weight as you want and also improve your overall health and life in the process.

The program is based on a revolutionary type of medicine known as functional medicine, and it works by addressing four major imbalances that are occurring in most modern Americans and keeping them overweight and functioning with less than optimal health.

WHAT IS FUNCTIONAL MEDICINE?

Functional medicine is an alternative branch of medicine that focuses on getting to the root causes of your symptoms (which includes excess body fat) using all natural techniques. Let me give you an example of how it differs from the type of practice most Americans are used to getting from their doctors.

Let's say you went to your current general practitioner, and you said you are having trouble keeping your weight down. You also mention you often feel bloated and gassy after eating, you're having trouble sleeping, your hair is starting to thin and you are more easily irritated these days.

Typically, your doctor would listen for a few minutes and then run some quick, basic tests. Afterward, he would give you a diagnosis that described your symptoms. For example, if you couldn't sleep, it would be insomnia. If your blood pressure was elevated, your diagnosis would be high blood pressure. And while these diagnoses are accurate descriptions of your symptoms, they don't say anything about what is actually causing them, do they?

The solution, according to mainstream medicine, is a cocktail of various expensive pharmaceutical drugs to quiet your symptoms. If you had further questions about your bloating, sleeping or irritability, your doctor would most likely provide referrals to numerous other specialists, or maybe tack on an extra prescription or two saying, "Try this and see if it works."

Trusting in your doctor, you start taking all of the drugs. After three months on all the prescribed drugs, your original symptoms have dulled a little, but they are still noticeable and prohibit you from living the life you really want. But now, in addition, you have developed other symptoms and side effects from all the harsh chemicals in your system.

Concerned, you go back to your doctor and tell him that none of your symptoms are completely healed, you even have a few new ones— and you are having a few strange reactions to the drugs. He takes some more quick tests and gives you a new cocktail of the latest, most promising drugs. Unfortunately, they don't ever get at the root cause either nor will they ever give you the optimal health you are seeking.

THE BIKINI CODE SPIRAL OF STRESS AND FAT JAIL

If you're honest with yourself, you can most likely recall a similar situation you or a loved one has been through. I call this deadly cycle of stress, disease and drug dependence the Bikini Code Spiral of Stress. I named it that because the stress of being overweight, sick, fatigued and constantly going from doctor to doctor, creates dozens of pressures that are constantly compounding and actually working against you and your health.

When this happens over time, all of those forces become so strong that you might feel like your health is spiraling out of control. I often hear patients say it feels like their health is circling the drain. You will learn throughout this book that chronic stress of any kind takes a heavy toll on your body and health. This is not a healthy way to live and is certainly not a path that will lead you to optimal health.

This Spiral of Stress causes millions of Americans to spend their entire lives taking potentially harmful, expensive and often-ineffective prescription drugs while never actually healing their bodies.

To top it all off, as part of this Spiral of Stress, your body creates what I call the Fat Jail. I call it that for two reasons. First, because you feel like you're in jail when you have excess weight and don't have the freedom to live the life you want to live. And second, because, what is jail? It is a storage unit for criminals. Well, the fat in your body is a storage unit for bad things, too. Fat stores many things. It stores fuel for your body, but it also stores chemicals (that I liken to criminals). So if you have a lot of chemicals and toxicity in your body from certain foods, prescription drugs and numerous other lifestyle choices, then they are naturally stored in your fat.

Further contributing to your Spiral of Stress and Fat Jail, this lifestyle does not afford you the energy or health to exercise. Most of the time, people who are stuck in the Spiral of Stress don't have the energy to move at the end of the day, much less work out. This only compounds the problem and makes trying to get healthy and happy even more frustrating. I have been in this maddening cycle. It is not fun, and it is virtually impossible to escape because you think you are doing yourself a favor by taking medications.

HOW IS FUNCTIONAL MEDICINE DIFFERENT?

For decades, you have been taught to trust and follow this symptom management and drug-based type medical care. But, there is another option. Let's pretend you took that same list of symptoms to a functional medicine physician. Here's how it probably would go

The very first thing the physician would do is give you a comprehensive health and life history survey that would include almost everything. These evaluations can reach 30 pages in length, and yes, we even care if you were breast or bottle-fed.

Then, based on your symptoms and history, the doctor would start a series of revolutionary tests designed to determine exactly how all your major biological systems (digestive, nervous, endocrine, immune, etc.) are functioning or not functioning. This way there is no generalizing or guessing as to what is wrong.

You will learn much more about these exciting tests in future chapters of the book, but the main thing to realize right now is that they are meant to find precise evidence of functionality issues occurring in your body on a cellular level.

Based on your test results, your doctor would then most likely discuss your diet with you in great detail as gastrointestinal health is at the core of this practice. All natural supplements, bio-identical hormones and detoxification methods would most likely round out your "prescription."

Functional medicine practitioners don't deny that antibiotics and other drugs and surgeries are appropriate and necessary in difficult and emergency cases. However, we do believe in using natural practices when at all possible. Our goal is to get you off chemical-based medications that can cause harm to your body. Using natural methods is only part of the backbone that supports functional medicine. The following are other key principles .

Based on Science

One of my favorite things about functional medicine is that it gets back to the basic science of health. Instead of just talking with patients about their symptoms, I now use scientifically advanced tests to detect extremely specific reactions that are occurring in the body and use the readings to accurately understand what is happening with patients on the most basic cellular level.

Holistic by Nature

Functional medicine is holistic, meaning it addresses the body as a whole and understands the importance of all the major biological systems working in harmony together, much like a city. As practitioners, we do not target just one symptom or disease; instead, we aim to heal all the working parts and dissolve any manifestation of poor health.

Going All-Natural

As I said earlier, we trust nature and believe in using all-natural remedies whenever possible. Our main tools are lifestyle management, nutritional guidance, proven natural supplements, bio-identical hormone therapies and emotional support toward a stress-free life.

Striving for Optimal Health

Functional medicine doesn't settle for average health. The purpose of the practice is to have all systems of the body working together to create overall, peak health and functionality.

Practicing Prevention

I have seen and experienced first-hand the infinite restorative and healing effects of this practice; but prevention is also one of its most important cornerstones. By regulating and monitoring the body's main functions and systems, patients can stave off every major disease that we currently face: heart disease, cancer, diabetes, auto-immune diseases, dementia and other mental illnesses.

WHO CAN BENEFIT FROM THE BIKINI CODE PROGRAM?*

Most of my patients come to me because they have heard that the Bikini Code program is guaranteed to help them naturally lose a significant amount of weight. And that is true. But weight is really just a symptom of poor health, and it is important to take inventory of all your health concerns if you really want to make a lasting, significant change because, as you will see, all of your symptoms are related to just a few core issues.

While some of the conditions below may be related to other serious health problems, many are related to the exact same issues that are causing you to gain weight. As you go through the list, please make a note where you see your symptoms.

Excess Body Fat

Many health authorities define weight problems using the following criteria: You are classified as overweight if your body mass index (BMI) is 25 to 29. You are considered obese if your BMI is between 30 and 39, and morbidly obese if it is above 40. Super obesity is anything higher than that. However, the truth is any extra weight is a sign that something is unbalanced in your body.

Fatigue

Chronic fatigue is characterized by an inability to feel refreshed upon awakening, feelings of extreme tiredness at inappropriate times during the day, fighting urges to sleep throughout the day, not having the energy and drive to complete tasks with the same levels of energy as you used to and avoiding certain situations because of lack of energy. It is considered chronic if symptoms last for over six months.

Insomnia

A broad term for a variety of sleep disturbances, but it is often defined as a difficulty falling or staying asleep that is not attributed to other medical or environmental causes, such as medication. It is usually considered a problem if this occurs for a month or more and causes significant distress in occupational, social or other important areas of function.

Irritable Bowel Syndrome (IBS)

Chronic constipation and recurrent diarrhea are both very common lower gastrointestinal problems. Both conditions are characterized by abdominal discomfort or pain relieved with defecation, and they are often associated with a change in frequency or appearance of stool. Symptoms may include fewer than three bowel movements per week, hard or lumpy stool or loose or watery stool, straining during a bowel movement or abdominal fullness and bloating.

Dyspepsia (heart burn)

An upper gastrointestinal condition that is most often associated with a burning sensation in the esophagus, excessive belching, fullness, gastric pain, nausea or vomiting after eating.

Mood Disturbances

Conditions that affect your general disposition and can include depression and extreme sadness, anxiety, mania, unstable emotions, irritability and anger issues. They often have a significant impact on your social and professional interactions.

Cognitive Disorders

Issues of brain function are often characterized by conditions like Attention Deficit Disorder (ADD), Attention Deficit and Hyperactivity

Disorder (ADHD), memory problems, difficulty concentrating, problems with rational thinking and lack of creativity.

Decreased Libido
A condition that affects both women and men and is characterized by a lack of interest in any sexual activity, not associated with one specific person or a severe arousal disorder. Symptoms include a general disinterest in sex (including masturbation) or a feeling like you could go the rest of your life without ever having sex.

Female Hormone Problems
Result in a variety of symptoms related to menstruation, perimenopause and menopause. Problems here are characterized by painful, heavy or irregular menstrual cycles, fibroids, endometriosis, decreased sex drive, mood disturbances, bloating and headaches.

Male Hormone Problems
Caused by a decrease in testosterone production. This condition is known as andropause and is characterized by weight gain, mood disturbances, sexual dysfunction and an overall lack of drive for life.

Hair, Skin, and Nail changes
Often overlooked as symptoms of health problems and widely thought of as superficial concerns. But the truth is acne, rapidly thinning and graying hair, thin and brittle nails and sallow skin are all indicators of imbalances inside your body.

Fibromyalgia/migraine headaches
Fibromyalgia is characterized by chronic, widespread abnormal pain that causes sleep disturbances, fatigue, stiffness in your joints, tingling or numbness, cognitive impairment and other pain symptoms. Migraine headaches are often associated with fibromyalgia but can occur on their own as well.

Frequent Illness
Results of a weakened immune system and can lead to frequent colds, sinus problems, infections, yeast infections and other illnesses. If you are getting sick numerous times throughout the year, there is a good chance that your immune system isn't functioning optimally, which is a result of a deeper imbalance.

THE BIG THREE: THE AMERICAN TRIOLOGY

The following three symptoms are so common and so harmful that they deserve their own category. Over half a million people die from heart disease every year. Below are the biggest factors and conditions that contribute to that number. I call them the American Trilogy because they are the culprits of this country's biggest health concerns.

High Blood Pressure

A condition when your blood flow creates unnecessary strain by pushing against your arteries, and it can damage your circulatory system in many ways. Chronic high blood pressure can lead to heart attacks and strokes. There are almost no symptoms associated with this condition, which is why it is often called the silent killer, but any physician can easily measure this with basic medical instruments.

Diabetes

Occurs when your body has become resistant to insulin. Diabetes can lead to blindness, kidney failure, heart attack, stroke and amputation of limbs. The symptoms vary but often include extreme thirst or hunger, weight gain, an inability to heal sores, fatigue and frequent urination.

High Cholesterol

Is virtually undetectable and void of symptoms. It is caused by the build-up of LDL (bad) cholesterol in the arteries and the deficiency of HDL (good) cholesterol.

*DISCLAIMER: The Cracking the Bikini Code program may help alleviate many of the symptoms described above, but it is in no way intended to replace medical treatment from a physician. In addition, those who are suffering from advanced diabetes, renal failure or are undergoing treatment for cancer should absolutely not attempt this program. You should always consult with your doctor about whether this, or any similar program is appropriate for you and how your current medications could be affected by a weight loss program of this nature.

BIKINI BODY BOTTOM LINE

Perhaps you recognize yourself in some of the descriptions above. I know when I was overweight I had many of them. I hope you did too because **Key #1 to Cracking the Bikini Code is to Be Honest About Your Health.**

This is important in terms of weight loss because you have to realize excess weight is only a sliver of the actual problem, and until you solve the whole puzzle, you will never achieve lasting health or weight management. By recognizing the other symptoms, you can start to put all the pieces of your complete health together to achieve permanent weight loss and to reach the dream life you envisioned at the beginning of the chapter. It can be yours.

But before we dive in, I want to give you a few more important words of encouragement. One of the best aspects of this program and this medicine is that if you follow the directions, you will succeed. I have never seen it fail when done correctly. That's why I encourage you to think of this book and program as your personal GPS system for getting to your dream life, health and body.

HOW LINDA S. CRACKED THE BIKINI CODE

At 38 years old, Linda came to me because she said her health and weight were spiraling out of control. She admitted that at certain times she felt like her overeating was uncontrollable, which contributed to her 55 pounds of excess body fat.

She blamed the excess weight for her low energy levels, which made everyday tasks, including performing at her job as a high school teacher or spending time with her family, a real struggle. On top of that, over the past few years her menstrual cycles had become increasingly more painful and irregular.

Like all of my patients, her physical appearance also spoke volumes about her health. The majority of her excess weight was located in her midsection, which caused her clothes to fit poorly and made her feel uncomfortable in social situations. Her eyes were lifeless, her skin sallow, fingernails thin and cracking, and her hair straw-like and brittle.

Even her personality suffered and she found herself short-tempered with co-workers and family members. She said the symptoms started after she gave birth to her last child about three years prior but progressed to unmanageable levels when her father died six months before she came to see me.

When I put Linda through Phase I of the Cracking the Bikini Code program, in the first six weeks her appetite subsided and she lost 31 pounds and began to sleep better. She also enjoyed increased energy levels, a restored sex drive and more regular, less painful cycles.

In Phase II, I found that she indeed had imbalances in all four of the major categories, but her hormone imbalance was particularly pronounced. Once we identified her exact hormone profile, we went about correcting all the imbalances. We were able to even out her hormone levels using natural supplements, bio-identical hormones, stress management tools and elimination tools for inflammation. We used bio-identical hormones to replace the progesterone her body was no longer making due to her age. This helped regulate her periods and render them less painful. These solutions, combined with nutritional guidance and detoxification efforts, produced results greater than she even hoped.

As she continued through Phase III of the program, she continued to lose about two pounds per week and eventually shed all of her excess weight. Her skin and hair started to look healthier, and she was able to take pride in her appearance for the first time in years. One of the greatest results was a better relationship with her friends and family. Her love of teaching also returned. She found her irritability significantly diminished, and she was able to enjoy life again.

TIPS FOR SUCCESS
[BE HONEST ABOUT YOUR HEALTH]

1. Question the status quo of the health care you're receiving.

2. Ask yourself: Are the prescription medicines I am taking (or have taken) really healing my symptoms or just masking them?

3. Be honest with yourself and your doctor. Don't edit your symptoms.

4. Ask lots of questions in regards to your health. Don't settle for an answer based on a pharmaceutical drug, unless the reasoning for a drug decision has been thoroughly explained and justified to you.

5. Understand that there is a natural way to lose weight, balance your body and achieve optimal health.

6. Take control of your own health. Don't expect your physician to be your champion. Spend time researching and exploring your own health and options.

CHAPTER 2
Inform Yourself

"A bikini is like a barbed-wire fence. It protects the property without obstructing the view."

— Joey Adams, actress

AFTER BEING HONEST WITH YOURSELF AND GOING through both the visualization and the self-evaluation exercises in Chapter 1, you now have two important things you need to start Cracking the Bikini Code. First, you have a clear vision of what your life would feel like with an ideal weight and optimal health. And second, you have a detailed picture of where your overall wellness is right now.

But the question still remains: What is the connection between your desired body and health and your actual body and health? Many women think, *If I just starve myself and eat a lot less, I will be thin*. Or, *If I kill myself at the gym six days a week, I could get the body I want*. And unfortunately, mainstream medicine encourages this behavior. If you told your physician you wanted to lose weight they would say, "Eat less. Move more." Right? Well, that's because they subscribe to the ancient idea that the body is like a bank: too much in, not enough out. When in reality, it is a complex bio-chemical equation.

Don't get me wrong, that advice is correct to an extent, as in exercise and a healthy diet are vital to good health, but they aren't the only factors. Functional medicine recognizes that if you have excess fat, there are complicated layers of other imbalances going on inside your body preventing you from living the life you want.

These layers are born out of four main imbalances. If they are present, no amount of dieting and exercise is going to help you long-term or make you feel truly balanced. This is why you must be informed about the truth behind your health and weight problems.

WHAT ARE THE FOUR IMBALANCES?

Most Americans consider weight gain an inevitable consequence of the aging process because for a long time we have accepted a slowing metabolism as a natural part of life. In the same vein, many people think chronic aches, pains and fatigue are just a part of growing older. But the truth is, they don't have to be. Everyone has the potential to live a full and vibrant life like the one you visualized in the beginning of Chapter 1.

This is a book primarily about weight loss, so that will be our focus as we go along. But you will come to see if you are suffering from excess weight, chances are you are also experiencing many other symptoms. And that's because all your health problems are connected and boil down to four major chronic imbalances. I will explore these symptoms in great detail throughout the book, but first I'd like to introduce the four major imbalances.

1. Hormone Imbalance

Your seven master hormones (cortisol, insulin, thyroid, DHEA, estrogen, progesterone and testosterone) govern almost every function in your body, including your metabolism. When they are imbalanced, they can wreak havoc on both your physical and mental health and make weight loss nearly impossible.

2. Toxicity Imbalance

The modern world is filled with toxic chemicals that when ingested or absorbed are stored in your fat and organ systems if not properly disposed of by your body. In addition, you manufacture a great deal of toxicity right in your own body. These toxins make it impossible for your organs and organ systems to function properly. The ability to recognize and rid your body of these toxins is crucial to optimal health and weight loss.

3. Nutrition Imbalance

The majority of Americans unknowingly suffer from serious nutritional deficiencies (despite being overweight), which cripple their health and keep them from living a life of vitality and health. Correction of these deficiencies allows for proper functioning of the body and alleviation of symptoms. Nutrition is also key to weight loss because you can't burn fat without certain nutrients.

4. Mental, Emotional and Spiritual Imbalance

Your health and weight are direct manifestations of your mental state. Your weight and body will never be truly optimal if you don't also address your mental, emotional and spiritual well-being.

That is a very brief introduction to the four imbalances. I have dedicated future chapters to each of the four imbalances, but it is important to start familiarizing yourself with them now.

WHY YOUR DOCTOR DOSEN'T TALK ABOUT THESE THINGS

The question patients ask most often is, "Why didn't my doctor tell me about these imbalances?" Having worked in mainstream medicine for 20 years, I can say without a doubt that mainstream doctors don't talk about these things because they are unaware of them; and they are unaware of them because there is no drug to fix it. In functional medicine, we harness your body's natural ability to heal itself through natural measures such as diet and nutritional supplementation. But in mainstream medicine, if there's not a quick-fix pharmaceutical drug, then you're not going to hear about it.

Unfortunately, this happens because pharmaceutical drug companies, with large advertising budgets and regular access to doctors by way of expert salespeople, actually dictate what goes on in mainstream medicine by informing both patients and physicians about the latest miracle drug. These same companies never look into funding research to heal these problems because the solutions are natural—which means they can't patent them, control the profit margin and make a lot of money.

It's not a pleasant way to look at our health care system, but unfortunately it is the truth. Big Pharma (my name for the industry as a whole) creates our expectations of what health care is in this country. It's a good thing there is another option. But, you need to inform yourself about other options because your regular physician will not.

HOW DO YOU KNOW IF YOU SUFFER FROM IMBALANCES?*

But how do you know if functional medicine can help you? Here is a shortened version of the questionnaire I give all my new patients. While it is important to realize that some of these symptoms may be caused by other conditions or diseases, they can often be indicators that you are experiencing one of the four imbalances I just mentioned. Please circle or highlight each symptom you are currently experiencing. If you check one or more boxes in a section, you may be experiencing an imbalance in that area.

QUICK CHECK: HORMONES

- Weight gain
- Irregular or heavy periods
- PMS or menopause symptoms
- Decreased sex drive
- Mood and memory problems (irritability, anxiety, depression)
- Less than one bowel movement daily
- Fatigue or insomnia
- Stressful lifestyle
- Frequent illness
- Foggy thinking
- Sugar cravings
- Consume sweet or starchy foods often

QUICK CHECK: TOXICITY

- Weight gain
- Mood and memory problems (irritability, anxiety, depression)
- Headaches
- Fatigue or insomnia
- Acne
- Frequent illness
- Skin, hair, nail issues
- Dark circles under eyes
- Joint or muscle pain
- Bowel problems (GERD, IBS, constipation, etc.)
- Ringing in ears
- Sinus problems

QUICK CHECK: MALNUTRITION

- Bowel problems (GERD, IBS, constipation, etc.)
- Recurrent yeast infections
- Sugar cravings
- Drink alcohol more than once weekly
- Antibiotic usage in the past two years
- Seasonal allergies or sinusitis
- Weight gain
- Mood and memory problems (irritability, anxiety, depression)
- Hair loss

QUICK CHECK: MENTAL, EMOTIONAL, SPIRITUAL

Mental
- Poor memory
- Lack of creativity
- Difficulty concentrating
- General dullness of the mind

Emotional
- Depression
- Anxiety, fear
- Frequent irritability
- Anger problems
- Unstable Emotions

Spiritual
- Low self-esteem
- Overall negative outlook on life
- Low drive for life
- Inability to see good things in your life
- Lack of respect for yourself or others

*DISCLAIMER: The Cracking the Bikini Code program may help alleviate many of the symptoms described above, but it is in no way intended to replace medical treatment from a physician. In addition, those who are suffering from advanced diabetes, renal failure or are undergoing treatment for cancer should absolutely not attempt this program. You should always consult with your doctor about whether this, or any similar program is appropriate for you and how your current medications could be affected by a weight loss program of this nature.

Visit truebalance.com for a more comprehensive inventory with scoring capabilities.

THE BIKINI CODE BREAKDOWN

The purpose of this questionnaire is to give you a reality check; it shows you that many of the discomforts in your life are actually indicators of deeper issues. If you are ready to start freeing yourself from some of these symptoms, read on.

This book is broken up into three parts. Part I focuses on education and information. You will learn the Six Keys to Cracking the Bikini Code, which explain how the program, using functional medicine practices, evaluates and treats your health and weight issues. What you read about this revolutionary science will enlighten you about what is actually going on inside your body on a cellular level and why you have not lost weight or achieved optimal health in the past.

Part II is a step-by-step guide that shows you how to incorporate these principles into your life so that you get balanced and lose weight once and for all. I take all the guesswork out of getting healthy.

Part III is a resource section that contains a recipe guide and suggested resource list. It is geared toward making the program as easy as possible for you. My goal here is to give you access to as many tools as possible to help you succeed.

BIKINI CODE BOTTOM LINE

I hope you are starting to see that while you may have thought you bought a diet book, what you actually got was a transformational tool kit that will not only change your health for life and help you get a bikini body, but it will also help you get to the life of your dreams. All these tools are given to you so that you can become familiar with what is going on inside your body. That is why **Key # 2 is to Inform Yourself About Your Body and Health.**

HOW KRISTEN BECAME TRULY BALANCED

Kristen was 42 years old when she cracked the Bikini Code. She was a wife and a mother of two. During her first pregnancy, she gained 30 pounds, which she lost easily afterward. During her second pregnancy, however, she gained a whopping 57 pounds and was not able to lose it all.

After her pregnancies, she gained another 40 pounds, especially in her midsection and developed problems sleeping. She also had no sex drive and was tired all the time. She said she felt like her body was controlling her life and had tried multiple programs to get herself back on track, but failed miserably each time.

Although weight was Kristen's biggest concern, she said she noticed other subtle symptoms occurring in her body. For example, she had increasing allergic symptoms, such as a chronic runny nose, itchy eyes, dark circles and puffiness under her eyes. To control the symptoms, she took allergy medicine regularly. She also experienced swelling in her hands and feet at the end of each day. To top it off, she only had one bowel movement every three to four days.

To remedy her symptoms, she started exercising and tried a whole slew of fad diets, but they got her nowhere. When she went to see her primary care doctor, he prescribed her the weight loss drug phentermine. He also gave her a diuretic for her swelling, a sleeping pill, allergy medicine, a stool softener with laxative to take daily and told her that the decreased sex drive was normal for her age. At first she lost a little weight, but she eventually gained it back and then some.

When she realized she was spending a fortune in co-pays at the pharmacy with very little results, she started questioning and researching the drugs she had been prescribed. She was appalled to learn about all of the potential side effects. In particular, it disturbed her to learn that the sleep aid was potentially addicting and could disrupt restorative sleep. That's when Kristen came to see me.

During our initial appointment, I listened to her fears and questions, and we discussed her concerns in detail. Eventually, I educated her about functional medicine and the four imbalances the program addresses. I showed her how her symptoms, which included weight gain, were all connected to the same core problems. I explained that the swelling, allergies, dark circles and constipation were all signs of toxicity and nutritional deficiencies. Her low sex drive and sleep problems spoke volumes about her hormone levels and mental, emotional and spiritual health.

Once she understood that she had been controlling symptoms with drugs and not fixing the root problems, a light bulb went off in her head, and she never went back. Kristen lost 22 pounds in the first six weeks (Phase I of the program) and all of her symptoms improved. During Phase II of the program, we found out she had severe food sensitivities, toxic yeast overgrowth (which you will learn about shortly) and significant magnesium deficiency, among other imbalances.

During this time, she also addressed the mental, emotional and spiritual part of the program. In doing so, she also admitted that she put her lifelong dream of becoming a nurse on the back burner to focus on her family. The suppression of her dreams was creating a frustration in her life that she had not previously recognized and certainly had never discussed with her regular doctor because he had never asked.

With the tools I gave her, Kristen understood exactly what to do *to make her feel better, and there was no stopping her. Her hormones balanced out, she detoxified, she nutrified and regained mental, emotional and spiritual balance. Her body responded beautifully, and she was ecstatic that now she controlled her body instead of the other way around. She also enrolled in nursing school to follow her passion, and that gave her an enormous, restored sense of confidence and happiness. Her two children and her husband enjoyed having their old Kristen back. Ultimately, she lost over 70 pounds and got off all the prescription medications that she had been given.*

Tips for Success
[INFORM YOURSELF]

1. Recognize that true optimal health and sustained weight loss cannot be achieved through cutting calories and exercise alone. There are many contributing factors.

2. Understand that mainstream medicine is based on drugs that rarely treat your underlying problem. Often times the drugs themselves are the cause of various symptoms, toxic buildup and health problems.

3. Learn that functional medicine specialized testing will identify factors contributing to your Spiral of Stress and Fat Jail.

4. Empower yourself with knowledge. Find out as much as you can about alternative options.

5. Don't expect that mainstream medicine will cure what ails you. It may make you feel better in the short term but ultimately it will never restore normal function, optimal health and longevity like functional medicine will.

CHAPTER 3

Keep Your Hormones Balanced

"Since the beginning, the bikini has represented freedom, fun and a sense of liberation."

— Malia Mills, fashion designer

N OW THAT YOU HAVE EVALUATED YOUR HEALTH, AND you have been informed about the four major imbalances, it is time to dig deeper into the science behind the program so that you understand what those imbalances mean for your health and weight. We will start with your hormones.

Your hormones function as one of your body's primary communication systems. They are produced by the endocrine system, which is made up of tiny glands all over your body that are all continuously secreting dozens of hormones into your bloodstream. Once in the bloodstream, these hormones become chemical messengers, acting like a wireless Internet communication system that sends signals and information all over your body.

The primary purpose of these signals is to communicate with each other and with your organ systems about what is going on inside your body. They share information about many processes but are primarily concerned with your body's energy production, metabolism regulation, tissue growth and development, mood regulation, sex drive and sleep patterns.

To help illustrate the vital importance of this communication system, imagine your body as your household. Your hormones are the wireless Internet connection. How do you think your family members would react if the connection became weak and faulty?

I know what would happen in my house. My teenage daughter would have a meltdown, stomp out of her room and start yelling about how she can't talk to her friends or surf the web. My son who loves video games would also get frustrated and angry, and within a very short time everyone would be complaining and unhappy. If this happened for a prolonged amount of time, this would also affect the professional and educational productivity of everyone in the household as no one could email or do research.

It is the same for your body. When your hormones are not functioning properly and doing their job, all of your biological systems get confused, out of sync and imbalanced. When they stay imbalanced for years on end, they get weak, taxed and start to fail. If the error in communication lasts for a prolonged amount of time, then significant damage to your health will occur. This damage includes weight gain, as your hormones primarily drive your metabolism. Similarly, if my kids never had Internet access they would go to their friends' houses, and our relationship would certainly suffer.

THE SEVEN MASTER HORMONES AND YOUR HEALTH

I believe that knowledge is power—especially when it comes to your health—so now that you have a general idea of how hormones act in your body, let's get a little more specific.

Your endocrine system is very intricate and produces lots of different hormones that all work together. But there are seven master hormones that I believe are the most significant.

You have probably heard of many of these hormones before, but there will also be some that are unfamiliar. And that's because your regular doctor and mainstream medicine don't talk about them. Why don't they talk about them? Like I said before, the reason is because there is no drug to treat a majority of hormone imbalances.

There are a few on the list that mainstream doctors say they test. I have patients tell me all the time, "My doctor tested my thyroid and it's fine." Despite their insistence, I find that 60 percent of these people have low thyroid.

Why? Well, that's because in functional medicine, we use different standards. Mainstream medicine practitioners tend to say hormone levels are fine as long as a disease has not developed yet. Whereas functional medicine practitioners know that if an organ or system isn't functioning at an optimal level, it is causing problems with your health. In addition, functional medicine compares your lab values with optimally healthy people, while mainstream medicine compares test results to the general population, which includes unhealthy people. I don't know about you, but I want my values compared to optimally healthy people because that's what I want for myself.

All that said, below is a list of your seven master hormones and a little about how, when imbalanced, they can keep you from achieving optimal health and your bikini body.

1. Cortisol

If there is one hormone that outranks the rest, it is cortisol. Cortisol is a regulatory steroid hormone triggered by stress (I'll define stress in just a moment). It is produced by your adrenal glands and is sometimes called the "fight, flight or freeze" hormone because when your body is under stress, your cortisol levels immediately increase due to issue dictums of your body's cells, telling them what to do and how to handle the problem. In short, it is the interface between stressors and your body.

It has long been understood that the human body produces cortisol as a defense mechanism to help us react to dangerous situations. Millions of years ago, these situations might have included a lion, bear or other predatory attack. And you might say, "Well, I don't have to worry about being attacked, so high levels of cortisol shouldn't affect me." But that assumption is incorrect.

In recent years, we've learned cortisol isn't just triggered in typical fight, flight or freeze moments. In fact, any and all types of stress send it soaring. It is a panic signal for the body whenever something is going wrong.

At first it sounds like a good thing, right? Well it is, except that due to the various demands of modern society, many Americans are walking around with extraordinary amounts of chronic stress, both mental and physical. This triggers an unnatural extended period of cortisol production, which taxes your body's energy resources.

But what is stress? When you first hear the word "stress" you most likely think about emotional and mental stresses like fear, anger, frustration, death, personal injury, job stress, moving, relationships, getting married, getting divorced, financial problems and so on. These are all very real stressors, and they do trigger cortisol production.

Just think back to the last time you said, "I am so stressed out!" Or the last time you got angry with a partner, boss or driver who cut you off in traffic. Your heart rate elevated, right? Your face might have flushed or you started to sweat. Cortisol was responsible for telling your body to have those reactions to the stressful situation.

You can probably easily identify those things in your life that cause mental stress. You can point to your boss, your bank account or your family. But I'm going to let you in on a big secret. There are many other things that are causing stress in your body and affecting your cortisol. These are things you may be totally unaware of because they are silently going on inside your body.

I'm talking about things like chronic inflammation of the gut from food sensitivities, early stages of various organ diseases, undiagnosed infections, chronic elevated blood glucose levels and detoxification issues. All of these problems cause internal stress on your body and, therefore, trigger cortisol production. We will get into many of those problems I just mentioned as we go along, but for now just remember that internal stress also causes your cortisol to spike.

If stressors, mental or physical, aren't removed and become a chronic problem, your body will struggle to keep up cortisol production. When you first start to experience chronic stress, your cortisol level rises to tell your cells to mobilize resources to deal with the stressor. And, cortisol is very good at its job. You typically go into a superwoman phase where you don't need a lot of sleep, you have a lot of energy and you are functioning super-normally. You can handle everything. Sounds good, right?

The problem is your body cannot maintain high levels of cortisol for extended periods of time. It depends on the stressor and the person as to what the reserves are; it could be days, it could be months or even years of stress before you start to see the effects. But eventually, these levels are going to start dropping. And once your cortisol starts dropping, it starts dropping in an irregular fashion. This is when you start getting tired in the morning. You don't want to get out of bed. You want to take a nap in the afternoon. You don't have energy. Or maybe you can't fall asleep or you fall asleep and wake up. Your energy levels become completely distorted.

If that continues and your levels go all the way down, you can develop adrenal fatigue syndrome, which is the medical term for what happens when your cortisol production becomes completely stressed out and can no longer function.

If your body is overproducing cortisol for too long or you develop adrenal fatigue, you will see all kinds of other imbalances and symptoms arise. This is primarily because all of your master hormone levels and your body's ability to produce them are interconnected. If your body is overproducing one, it is doing so at the cost of another hormone. Essentially, it's robbing Peter to pay Paul.

In particular, high cortisol levels draw heavily from your insulin and thyroid production, which creates all sorts of symptoms and diseases, including weight gain.

2. Insulin

Speaking of insulin, it is your second master hormone, and it is directly tied to your cortisol as well as your weight and metabolism. Its primary function is to regulate your blood sugar. So what does that mean? Well, all foods and beverages that you consume contain glucose (the scientific word for sugar). Some are obviously higher in sugar than others, but all foods have some. The glycemic index (GI) is a measurement of the amount of sugar in a food. Every food has a number, from 1 to 100, that signifies how much a food will increase your blood sugar after you consume it.

After you eat, glucose is released into your blood. If the food is high in sugar, your body produces higher levels of insulin to return your blood sugar to normal levels. It does this because your body likes your blood sugar level in a very narrow range, similar to how you like the temperature gauge in your car, right in the middle of too hot and too cold. Your body is picky about its glucose levels because going both too high and too low can be extremely harmful to your health.

So if you eat something with a low GI, like broccoli, there will be a small bump in your sugar levels and insulin production will be minimal. But if you eat something with a high GI, like a pastry, your levels will become quite high, and your body is going to have to work hard to produce insulin to bring it back down.

In addition to triggering cortisol production due to the stress it creates, when your blood glucose is chronically high, your insulin production also gets taxed and weak. If this becomes chronic, eventually when you eat a pastry and your blood glucose goes up, your system becomes unresponsive. This is called insulin resistance, and it is the precursor to diabetes and many other diseases.

Insulin problems are detrimental to your weight because if you cannot handle the heavy blood sugar load, the excess glucose has to go somewhere. Where does it go? Two places. First, it sticks to cells in your body and damages them. If you have sugar sticking to your cells it prohibits them from functioning optimally. And secondly, it is stored as fat. Neither option is good for you or your weight.

Because of the Standard American Diet (SAD), a very large portion of the general population has a sugar problem. Insulin and sugar problems can lead to obesity, diabetes, blindness, kidney failure, heart disease and attacks, dementia, stroke and weight gain. This is just one of the many reasons why diet is crucial to this program and to functional medicine as a whole. As you can see already, what you put in your mouth immediately affects your master hormones.

3. Thyroid

Your third master hormone is your thyroid hormone. It is number three on the list because it interacts with and is heavily affected by both cortisol and insulin. Your thyroid gland is a small butterfly-shaped organ located in your neck that largely regulates energy metabolism and distribution. It dictates how much energy needs to be burned by your different cells and how much needs to be stored in—you guessed it—fat. So it should be no surprise that when it is imbalanced you gain weight and suffer from other symptoms such as constipation, hot and cold sensitivities, hair loss, brittle nails and even insomnia.

The most common causes of a sluggish thyroid are chronic high cortisol and insulin levels. Your body's thyroid levels will decrease in response to chronically elevated cortisol and insulin levels. While it is a good checks-and-balances system in theory, when chronic stress exists, resources get tapped out quickly and thyroid production also becomes taxed and weak. If your levels become too low for too long, it is called hypothyroidism and it affects your entire body.

Like I said before, I see a lot of people who say their regular doctor checked their thyroid levels, and they were told that they are fine. But then they come to me, and I find out their thyroid is in fact sluggish. Does that mean that you have a thyroid disease? No. But it does mean your thyroid isn't functioning optimally, and it will show itself in a myriad of symptoms such as fatigue, constipation and weight gain.

4. DHEA (Dehydroepiandrosterone)

A complex hormone with many duties. But one of its main functions is to be your body's first safeguard against abnormal cortisol production. When your body triggers the production of cortisol it also produces DHEA, which can be converted into cortisol (many hormones have this morphing capability). Again, at first this seems like a great way to prevent a cortisol spiral, but it gets to be a real problem when it happens repeatedly.

The problem occurs because another main function of DHEA is to be the precursor hormone to all three of your sex hormones (estrogen, progesterone and testosterone). But if your body is forced to use all its DHEA to keep cortisol levels in check and deal with stress, it creates imbalances with your sex hormone production. This also results in weight gain, low sex drive, menstrual cycle issues and mood problems.

This is just another example of how all of your hormones are in a constant dance with each other. If you throw one off, the whole group will be off. Also, recognize that because all of these hormones directly affect your metabolism, keeping them balanced is crucial to weight management and bikini body success.

5, 6 & 7: The Sex Hormones: Estrogen, Progesterone & Testosterone

I group all of these hormones together because they define our physical sex characteristics and reproductive capacity. They greatly influence each other and small chemical reactions can turn one into the other.

Mainstream medicine treats them like silos—like one doesn't have anything to do with the other. But they have everything to do with each other. Proper levels of all of these confer a normal menstrual cycle and fertility in women. And, along with testosterone, they help to maintain many things, not only weight but mood and memory functions and sex drive.

As I mentioned earlier in this chapter, DHEA is a precursor to all of your sex hormones. But, DHEA is also the back-up system for low cortisol levels, meaning healthy levels of your sex hormones are entirely dependent on a normal production of all your other master hormones, especially cortisol. If those top four hormones are not balanced, neither are your sex hormones. This means that what you eat can affect your sex drive and menstrual cycle.

A COMPREHENSIVE CHECK: WHAT DOES A HORMONAL IMBALANCE LOOK LIKE?*

As I said, the only real way to really know if you have a hormonal imbalance is to get properly tested by a functional medicine practitioner. However, there are some telltale signs that can help you detect significant issues. Please check the following symptoms you are currently experiencing:*

Adrenal and Stress Hormones (cortisol)
• Fatigue or daytime sleepiness
• Difficulty falling, staying asleep

- Irritability, anxiety, depression
- Concentration, memory problems
- Weight gain
- Hair loss
- Salt cravings
- Drink caffeinated beverages more than twice weekly
- Drink alcohol more than once weekly
- Ringing in ears
- Swelling in extremities
- High stress job, relationship or life issues
- Chronic steroid use
- Abnormal reactions to medications
- High blood pressure
- Diabetes
- Arthritis
- Muscle pain or fibromyalgia
- Colitis or diverticulitis
- Autoimmune disease
- Sinusitis, allergies or asthma
- Chronic fatigue syndrome

Sex Hormones
- Irregular or heavy cycles
- PMS symptoms
- Fibroids, endometriosis, ovarian cysts
- Polycystic Ovarian Syndrome
- Infertility
- Fibrocystic breasts
- Breast or uterine cancer
- Menopause
- Hot flashes or night sweats
- Decreased sex drive
- Vaginal dryness
- Difficulty falling, staying asleep
- Daytime sleepiness or fatigue
- Headaches
- Irritability, anxiety, depression
- Concentration, memory problems
- Loss of muscle mass

- Acne
- Facial or excess body hair
- Hair loss

Thyroid Hormones
- Fatigue or daytime sleepiness
- Weight loss or gain
- Irritability, anxiety, depression
- Less than one bowel movement daily
- Loose or unformed stools
- Hair loss
- Palpitations
- Bulging eyes
- Dry skin or hair
- Cold hands or feet
- Cold intolerance
- Profuse sweating
- Thyroid disorder

Glucose and Insulin Hormone
- Weight gain
- Being overweight
- Inability to lose weight
- Fatigue
- Foggy thinking
- No regular exercise
- Sugar cravings
- Consume sweet drinks often
- Consume starchy foods often
- Eat dessert often
- Insulin resistance, pre-diabetes, or diabetes
- Thirst or excess urination

*DISCLAIMER: The Cracking the Bikini Code program may help alleviate many of the symptoms described above, but it is in no way intended to replace medical treatment from a physician. In addition, those who are suffering from advanced diabetes, renal failure or are undergoing treatment for cancer should absolutely not attempt this program. You should always consult with your doctor about whether this, or any similar program is appropriate for you and how your current medications could be affected by a weight loss program of this nature.

HOW DOES THE BIKINI CODE PROGRAM ADDRESS HORMONE IMBALANCES?

If you checked even one or two of those symptoms, there's a good chance you are experiencing a hormonal imbalance. Again, this doesn't mean you necessarily have a hormone disease. It just means that you are not functioning at an optimal level. And I would bet my bank account that you are having a hard time losing weight because of it.

So how do you heal an imbalance? Functional medicine addresses hormone imbalances in a few different ways: nutritional guidance, all-natural supplementation and, in some cases, bio-identical hormone therapies. Bio-identical hormones are not synthetic or animal hormones, like many of the hormone-related products, including birth control pills and shots, currently on the pharmaceutical market.

Bio-identical hormones are made in a lab, but they are created to mimic the exact hormones already found in your body. They work seamlessly with your body's natural hormone production. In Part II of the book, I will explain all these treatments in more detail and show you how I integrate them into the program.

BIKINI CODE BOTTOM LINE

Now you know the science behind **Key No. 3 to Cracking the Bikini Code: Keep Your Hormones Balanced**, but don't worry, there's not a quiz at the end of this book. The biggest thing I want you to take away from this chapter is that you have seven master hormones all working together as an integrated system to make sure your body is communicating and functioning optimally. When this system becomes stressed, it creates weight gain and disease, and communication breakdowns most often occur due to a few key things: external stress, internal inflammation due to gastrointestinal issues (more on this in Chapter 4) and chronic high blood sugar.

HOW SARAH CRACKED THE BIKINI CODE

Sarah was one of my youngest patients. At 16 years old, she was 30 pounds overweight and was prescribed birth control pills for three years to ease her extremely painful periods. She was a beautiful girl but obviously unhappy in her own skin and body. Aside from her weight, her list of symptoms included acne, chronic constipation and polycystic ovarian syndrome (PCOS). She also said she felt a great deal of shame for not looking like "normal" girls her age, which caused her to miss out on many social activities.

Because she was on birth control pills for so long, I knew a lot of what she was experiencing was related to hormone imbalances. After undergoing salivary hormone testing, we found that she had an excess of estrogen relative to her progesterone, which explained her PCOS. I knew immediately we had to detox the excess estrogen. Because she was still young, there was no need for her to go on bio-identical hormones; we removed a majority of the problem by changing her diet to get rid of all the estrogen-like compounds (caffeine, preservatives, other chemicals, and even flimsy plastic water bottles that leach chemicals into the water). On top of modifying her diet, I gave her natural supplements to help detoxify excess estrogen through the liver and support progesterone manufacture.

As a teenager, at first she struggled with giving up certain foods her friends were able to eat and initially felt frustrated. But after noticing significant results in her weight and skin in just the first few weeks, she decided to stick with the program. After going through the first two phases of the program, she lost all 30 pounds and was ecstatic with her new body shape. Her skin also cleared up and her periods became regular, allowing her to get off birth control for good.

Tips for Success:
[KEEP YOUR HORMONES BALANCED]

1. Understand hormones are like your body's wireless network. If your cells get out of touch with each other and are not functioning normally, then sustainable weight loss and optimal health is virtually impossible.

2. Cortisol is the cornerstone of your overall weight and well-being. Mainstream medicine generally does not address this because there is no drug to treat it.

3. Recognize stress comes in three forms: psychosocial, blood sugar imbalance and inflammation, all of which raise your cortisol levels. Eliminating stress of all kinds is key to keeping your hormones balanced and getting your bikini body.

4. What you eat not only affects your insulin and puts you at risk for diabetes, but it also directly affects your cortisol, and therefore everything else.

5. Don't think you can optimize health and lose weight without hormone regulation.

6. Taking birth control only masks your symptoms.

7. Imbalanced sex hormones create symptoms including decreased sex drive, painful periods and erectile dysfunction, but they can be addressed with natural measures such as diet modification.

Once you have reached this precarious state, your body is going to need a lot of repair to get your cortisol levels balanced again. But the good thing is once you know, you can start eliminating these stressors one by one.

In future chapters, I'm going to show you exactly how to eliminate stressors so you can get your communication system functioning properly.

CHAPTER 4
Illuminate & Eliminate Toxins In Your Life

"The sight of the first woman in the minimal two piece was as explosive as the detonation of the atomic bomb by the U.S. at Bikini Island in the Marshall Isles, hence the naming of the bikini."

— Tom Waits, singer-song writer, actor

THE SECOND OF THE FOUR MAJOR IMBALANCES AFFECTING most modern women is a buildup of harmful toxins in your body. Toxins are unnatural and harmful substances that contaminate your body from both internal sources (most likely your gastrointestinal tract) and external sources (various facets of your environment). Many of us don't realize how many toxins are affecting us on an every day basis or how harmful they can be. But the truth is detoxifying is essential in this day and age. Let me share a story with you to help illustrate the point.

Nicole was a patient of mine who up until recently was living a double life. On the outside, she was a successful business executive in her mid-forties, with an exciting job that took her all over the world. She loved her job immensely and was highly respected by her colleagues. She also had a healthy social life, with many friends and a caring husband. Many of her nights were filled with decadent dinners or cocktail parties, which she loved, despite the fact that she credited all that eating and drinking to her 35-pound weight gain.

Inside, however, Nicole was a mess. Her health was in serious trouble. For over ten years, she had struggled with a variety of issues concerning her gastrointestinal tract. These symptoms included severe bloating and gas, a bleeding rectum, stomach pain, and bouts of constipation and diarrhea. No one she worked with knew she was in pain or the great lengths she took to hide it. Completely embarrassed by it, she never complained or told people when she was going to the doctor. Her husband was the only one who knew about it, but even he didn't know just how bad it was.

Just a few months prior to coming to see me, her health took a turn for the worse. Her symptoms became severe and traveling became a major problem. She no longer felt that long flights or car rides were feasible or safe. If she couldn't find help quickly, she would be forced to resign from her job. While devastated about the prospect of giving up her job, she also worried about what she would tell people. Was she supposed to tell her peers that at 47 years old she often had to wear adult diapers and could no longer travel?

Over the years, she went to a few different gastroenterologists, and received diagnoses for everything from irritable bowel syndrome to gastritis (heartburn) to colitis. She had been tested for cancer numerous times, but the tests came back negative. Her doctors gave her prescriptions and said they would continue to watch her progress. Her symptoms got a little better with medication, but, inevitably, because they weren't getting at what was causing all these symptoms, problems still cropped up.

Finally, frustrated after years on drugs that didn't heal her, Nicole gave up all medication. That's when things got really bad. Her symptoms became out of control, and she thought resignation was the only option. Her doctor's answer was to put her on steroids and a bevy of potentially toxic medications.

As a last resort, she came to see me. She admitted she was skeptical of my system, but that she knew in her gut (pun intended) that prescription medicine and mainstream doctors were not actually helping her. So I evaluated her using functional medicine laboratory tests. What I found (and suspected from the time I first met Nicole) was that her gut was toxic. Her entire gastrointestinal tract, from her throat to her rectum, was literally on fire. My job was to figure out what was feeding this fire.

WHAT IS TOXICITY AND INFLAMMATION?

I'm sure you know the symptoms of a sinus infection: you feel like you have a fire in your face; your nose is red and hot, and you have swollen tissue in the face and throat, plus puss excretion—not fun. That is inflammation. It is a symptom of your immune system, which is like your body's military, attacking or protecting you from something that is toxic (bacteria in this case).

But just like a fire gives off toxins into the environment, the inflammation in your body (whether it is in your nose or your gut) gives off toxic chemical by-products into your bloodstream. These chemical by-products can wreak havoc on your body in many ways. Not only do they cause you to gain weight, but they also contribute to intestinal disorders, arthritis, fibromyalgia and other symptoms.

Like millions of Americans, due to her toxic diet and lifestyle, Nicole was experiencing chronic inflammation throughout her entire gastrointestinal tract. You can experience toxic build up and inflammation in many of your organs and organ systems. But your kidneys, liver, fat tissue, central nervous system and endocrine (hormones) systems are particularly affected.

This is why one of the primary concerns in functional medicine is detoxification, and **Key No. 4 is Illuminate and Eliminate Toxins In Your Life**. Eliminating toxins will help all of your organs function on a much higher level and reduce deadly chronic stress from inflammation.

When Nicole finally eliminated all the toxins from her life and worked toward naturally healing her gut, she completely resolved all of her gastrointestinal issues. And she didn't have to quit her job. While not everyone has symptoms like Nicole's, toxicity issues can present themselves in a variety of symptoms such as acne, insomnia, emotional problems, weight gain, fatigue and more.

WHAT CAUSES TOXICITY?

Unlike a sinus infection, which is caused by bacteria that can be killed to alleviate the symptoms, the majority of inflammation occurring in modern Americans is in the gut.

Inflammation of the gut is especially serious because it causes your cortisol levels to increase (thus creating problems with your other hormones) and prohibits your intestines from properly absorbing the nutrients you get through your diet. But possibly the worst complication of a chronically inflamed gut is the possibility of creating what functional medicine calls a leaky gut.

Leaky gut is when the lining of your gastrointestinal track gets so weak and worn down that it actually becomes permeable and small molecules of food leak out into your body. Of course, your body sees these molecules as foreign objects and attacks them, creating even more stress and inflammation in your body.

But the good news is that by choosing what goes into your body and what doesn't, you are able to naturally heal and resolve this problem. The usual suspects when it comes down to severe toxicity in the gut are broken down into four categories: food and drink items you ingest, pharmaceutical drugs, gastrointestinal infections and environmental issues.

1. Harmful Foods and Drinks

Food and water are the basic necessities of life, right? Yes, but they are also the number-one way to cause harm to your gastrointestinal tract. Here are three things to watch for when choosing what you are going to put into your body.

Unfriendly Foods

Did you know we are not supposed to eat the same foods every day? Or that based on your individual genetic lineage, lifestyle habits and body composition there are foods your body finds unfriendly? These are called food sensitivities, and if ignored, they will inflame, irritate and destroy your gut.

I'm not talking about true food allergies like peanuts or iodine or shellfish, where you eat it and your throat closes up and you could die. That's a true allergy. I'm talking about a sensitivity, where a different branch of your immune system reacts to certain foods that you eat and creates much less obvious—but still serious—symptoms. In functional medicine, one of the cornerstone tests is a food sensitivity test that will check your body's specific reaction to over 350 foods.

Chemically Processed Foods and Drinks

But unfortunately, food sensitivities are not all your gut is fighting. In addition, the modern Standard American Diet (SAD) is filled with packaged and processed foods that are saturated with chemicals, preservatives, food colorings and additives that your body recognizes as toxic. These toxins not only contribute to the destruction of the delicate lining of your gastrointestinal tract, but they significantly contribute to your weight because your body is unable to eliminate all of these harmful substances, so it stores them in fat. Hence the Fat Jail from Chapter 1.

Woeful Water

Water is essential. You drink it, cook with it, clean with it, brush your teeth with it and bathe in it. Tap water comes to your house in great abundance, and unless there is a drought, you probably use it in great volume on a daily basis without much thought. But did you ever stop to think about what exactly is in your water? That maybe all that water is contributing to your symptoms? Probably not.

As I mentioned before, I grew up in a pre-war building in Manhattan. It was filled with lead pipes. Of course, growing up I didn't really think twice about the water I was drinking, but years later when I tested myself for heavy metal toxicity (another cornerstone test for functional medicine), I found out that the cumulative effect was extraordinary. I had extremely high levels of lead and mercury in my blood stream, which are known to cause memory and mood problems, among other health issues.

But, it's not just heavy metals. Other toxins such as fluoride (yes, it is extremely bad for you, despite what your dentist has been telling you) reside in your tap water. And, just like the toxins from food, these foreign substances are often stored in your cells, fat tissue and other organs.

2. Dangerous Drugs

Yes, it is true that mainstream prescription drugs can quickly alleviate (although not always heal) pain and discomfort. But because they are comprised of unnatural compounds made by scientists in a lab, they leave behind all sorts of chemicals in your system.

Many of these toxic chemicals have profoundly negative effects on your body. For example, just a single round of antibiotics is enough to destroy most of the good bacteria that resides in your gastrointestinal tract, which helps you break down foods. It can take two years for good bacteria to return to normal levels. These bacteria keep you healthy and you could not live without them.

The goal of functional medicine is to get you off most, if not all, prescription drugs. If you take the time to heal your body naturally, you will be amazed at how many of those toxic and costly drugs you can stop taking.

3. Infections

Unfortunately, when addressing toxicity, your gut takes a lot of major hits. Not only is it responsible (along with the liver and kidneys) for processing the foods and drugs you put into your body, but also because it is a warm, moist environment with plenty of food, it is also a fertile breeding ground for parasites, harmful bacteria and yeast overgrowth. These often-undiagnosed foreign invaders further contribute to the degradation of your digestive system. In functional medicine, we use a stool evaluation to test for parasites and infections, such as round worms and hook worms, as well as for pathologic bacteria and yeast.

Overproduction of yeast is one of the most common problems we find. Yeast overgrowth is an opportunistic infection, and the top three issues that cause it are a diet rich in sugar (the primary food source for yeast), birth control pills and other prescribed daily drugs, and antibiotics.

All of these different pathogens are very stressful to your system, causing a weakened immune system, severe inflammation of the gastrointestinal tract, and destruction of the lining of your gut. In turn, these factors raise your cortisol level, which creates chaos all over your body.

Mainstream doctors sometimes test for these pests, but they do so by taking your stool, putting it under the microscope and reviewing it with the naked eye. However, it is a notoriously unpredictable test because it relies on the human eye to detect the presence of bugs. The functional medicine test is a DNA probe. It looks for the genetic material of the pathogen. So if it is there, we are going to find it. It is an extremely accurate test.

But why are these infections such a big deal? All of these bugs irritate your gut, but also they make toxic byproducts that go all over your body. Your body only has so much it can do to get rid of those chemicals. So guess what your body does with the excess toxins? Like everything else, it stores them in fat.

4. Environmental Issues

Food, water and pharmaceutical drugs are major contributors to toxic build up, and we are absorbing chemicals from all around us. The makeup you wear, the cleaning products you use in your house, the lotions and toothpaste you use, even your laundry detergent, are all being absorbed into your body and must be processed in some way. While I don't encourage my patients to become obsessive, it is very important to consider the substances you ingest, absorb and breathe every day.

A COMPREHENSIVE CHECK:
WHAT DOES A TOXCITY ISSUE LOOK LIKE?*

- Reaction to any food
  (gas, bloating, sinus blockage and stuffy nose)
- Reaction to smoke, perfume or other odors
- Skin rashes or hives
- Seasonal allergies or sinusitis
- Asthma or other respiratory disease
- Frequent infections or illnesses
- Autoimmune disease
- Inflammatory disease
- Arthritis
- Weight gain
- ADD/ADHD
- Concentration or memory problems
- Hair loss

*DISCLAIMER: The Cracking the Bikini Code program may help alleviate many of the symptoms described above, but it is in no way intended to replace medical treatment from a physician. In addition, those who are suffering from advanced diabetes, renal failure or are undergoing treatment for cancer should absolutely not attempt this program. You should always consult with your doctor about whether this, or any similar program is appropriate for you and how your current medications could be affected by a weight loss program of this nature.

HOW DOES THE BIKINI CODE PROGRAM
ADDRESS TOXICITY?

If you are not aware of how your body is processing toxins, you might end up in a situation like Nicole from the beginning of the chapter—miserable, embarrassed and in pain.

Luckily, Nicole came to see me, and I knew exactly what was happening. After changing her diet, putting her on a regimen of herbal detoxification supplements, eliminating the offending items in her life (gluten was a main culprit) and working to reduce as much of the inflammation in her gut as possible, Nicole was happily able to continue on with her life and career. She is able to travel now with confidence. But traveling isn't the only source of her confidence these days because while her toxin and digestive issues brought her to me, she lost 40 pounds in the process.

And it's no different for anyone else. Diet, herbal supplements and total elimination of toxins, sensitivities and infectients are the main ways in which functional medicine heals inflammation.

BIKINI CODE BOTTOM LINE

In 2014, if you're not detoxifying you're not going to achieve optimal health. Detoxification is crucial to both healthy function of all your organs and weight management.

HOW YOLANDA BECAME TRULY BALANCED

Yolanda was 42 years old and severely obese at 87 pounds overweight when she came to me. Although it didn't stop her from regularly overeating, she was suffering many symptoms associated with her digestive system. Her complaints included chronic constipation, bloating after eating and uncontrollable cravings for sugars and carbohydrates. She also admitted that she often had to take laxatives just to have a bowel movement and often went up to a week without one at all. In addition, she also mentioned that she suffered from chronic sinus congestion and infections (for which she had taken numerous rounds of antibiotics each year) and that her periods were often painful and uncomfortable. She also revealed scaly, itchy patches of skin (called psoriasis) that had recently cropped up in various places on her body.

Headaches and a general sense of foggy brain rounded out her extensive list of complaints.

All of these problems caused her to have an overall bloated appearance that included heavy bags under her eyes, swollen sinus cavities, and excess weight all over her body.

When I put Yolanda through the program, I found many imbalances and problems, but one major culprit: yeast overgrowth due to the large amount of sugar that was in her diet. This caused not only the yeast to take up residence but prohibited the good intestinal bacteria from being able to live. This combination had wreaked havoc on her entire gastrointestinal tract and was the root of a lot of her problems. I knew we had to break the cycle and get her off these sugary, nutrition- ally deficient foods.

In Phase I she initially struggled with the diet and suffered many carbohydrate cravings, so I placed her on natural carb-craving reducing supplements, which did the trick. Once we got her off the blood sugar roller coaster, her cravings stopped after the first week, and I was able to correct her blood sugar levels. In Phase I, she lost 33 pounds, and had bowel movements every day. Then, in Phase II she lost the remaining 54 pounds. Now she's in Phase III and has maintained her ideal body weight, which at 5' 4" is 125 pounds. In addition, her energy is better, her skin cleared up and she no longer needs medicated creams, and all the bloating went away. She is also now off the road to diabetes.

Tips for Success
[ILLUMINATE & ELIMINATE TOXINS IN YOUR LIFE]

1. Getting rid of all toxins is vital to getting a bikini body.

2. Eat all organic, fresh foods when at all possible. Avoid processed foods at all costs.

3. Thoroughly evaluate every single product you bring into your home and put into or on your body.

4. Do not let mainstream medicine doctors convince you that toxic prescription medicines are harmless or are the only option for treatment.

5. It is important to get a proper water filter. Plastic water bottles leach chemicals into the water that contribute to toxic buildup.

6. Recognize that much of the toxicity that affects your health comes from seemingly harmless foods that may be a staple in your diet and from gastrointestinal infections that mainstream medicine will routinely fail to diagnose and treat.

CHAPTER 5
Nutrify Your Body Properly

"I thought, If I'm so afraid of a bikini, there's something wrong. And so I had to get back into one."

— Valerie Bertinelli, actress

O FTEN TIMES WE ASSOCIATE MALNUTRITION (WHICH IS the third imbalance) with starving children in foreign countries. But would it shock you if I told you that the average American suffers from malnutrition, even if they are overweight and get more than three meals a day? I remember when I was overweight I actually thought that I had better nutrition than most other people. After all, I ate more than most people I knew. How could I be lacking anything? But, I could not have been more wrong. Throughout this chapter, you will learn why.

Chronic malnutrition is a problem that affects millions of people in America. In my practice, about 90 percent of my patients suffer from nutritional deficiencies and experience significant symptoms as a result. Mainstream medicine doesn't recognize it as a problem because the majority of people suffering from malnutrition in this country don't look like the emaciated children you see on TV ads. Additionally, once again, there is not a prescription drug that can help, so it is rarely discussed within the healthcare system with the proper depth and attention it deserves.

THE NUTRITION AND WEIGHT LOSS CONNECTION

Getting proper nutrition is a huge deal when it comes to your weight and health. Why? Because nutrients are the fuel for your cells and give them the energy necessary to complete virtually every function—including burning fat. But your body is like a highly advanced, finicky sports car. Not just any fuel will do. Your body must get enough high quality fuel in order to perform optimally.

To help you better understand what is proper fuel, here is a rundown of the basic building blocks of good nutrition and how they contribute to your bikini body (or lack thereof).

THE BIKINI BODY BUILDING BLOCKS

There are two major groups of nutrients: macronutrients and micronutrients. Macronutrients (macro meaning big) make up the majority of foods and are primarily used for energy production and metabolism. Micronutrients (micro meaning small) make up a very small—but integral—part of your diet, and aid in hormone production among other things. You should regard any "food" that doesn't fall into one of these categories (i.e. preservatives, pesticides, fillers, etc.) as toxins.

1. What are Macronutrients?

There are three basic essential macronutrients: carbohydrate, protein and fat. These are what give you the calories that your body uses to make adenosine triphosphate (ATP), the energy currency for your cells. Each molecule of ATP is like a dollar bill that a cell can "spend" to perform an action. But, within each category there are many different variations, some of them good for your health, and some of them extremely harmful.

Carbohydrates Can Be Your Friend

Due to fad diets like the Atkins Diet and other low-carb, high-protein diets, carbohydrates have a bad rap in this country. Many people believe in order to lose weight you have to eliminate all carbs from your diet for good. But the truth is some carbs can be a good fuel source in moderation and can help aid in weight loss. The key is to remember not all carbs are created equal.

Step away from simple carbs. Simple carbohydrates are also known as simple sugars, because they are in large part nothing but glucose. These are things like candy, cookies, bread, white potatoes, pasta, white rice and other starchy foods, like corn. These foods are quickly and easily absorbed into the blood stream.

They are often tasty, yes, but they cause your blood sugar levels to spike quickly, and remember what happens then: insulin problems, raised cortisol and weight gain. Everyone, and I mean everyone, should stay away from as many simple carbohydrates as possible. This may be hard at first because you have trained your taste buds to crave these things, but don't worry, you can retrain them with time.

Complex carbohydrates, on the other hand, are the true power-houses of energy. Unlike simple carbohydrates, they are not easily broken down and absorbed by your body. So your digestive system takes a while to break them down, releasing energy at a much slower pace. This gives you a sustained flow of energy, keeps your insulin at a good level, and helps you feel full longer. Complex carbohydrates are found mostly in vegetables, whole grains, beans, and nuts. Another great thing about complex carbs is they are often high in fiber, which helps clean out the all-important gastrointestinal tract.

Ultimately, the majority of your diet—about 60 percent—should come from this one type of macronutrient. I believe it is important to be informed about these foods, but please remember that I have included a diet guide for you at the end of this book, so try not to feel overwhelmed about all the specifics.

It Takes Fat to Burn Fat

Low-fat is considered a bad word in functional medicine. As with carbohydrates, the national media and health care providers have for years produced consumer propaganda crucifying fats. They asserted that fat makes you fat, so the mainstream idea was to eliminate all fat from your diet. In the 80s and 90s "low-fat" and "light" were key words in selling any food product. But the truth is that certain essential fats, such as omegas 3 and 6 are crucial to weight loss and health optimization. Good fats are the second best fuel source for your body. But, again like carbs, not all fats are created equal. There are some real killers out there. Here's the fat breakdown.

Unsaturated fats are found in foods like nuts and seeds, fish, avocados and olive oil. These are essential for many of your body's functions and are the best kind of fats for your body. When consumed on a regular basis, they can have great effects on your brain function, metabolism, hair, skin and nails and immune system.

Essential fatty acids are important fats that you must get through your diet. The two most important essential fatty acids are omega-3 and omega-6 fatty acids. These fats are very important for brain function, decreasing inflammation, lowering blood pressure and adrenal support. The best sources for these fats are fish, nuts, seeds and lamb. A deficiency in fatty acids can cause skin and hair problems, inflammation, mood and memory problems and immune system issues.

Saturated fats are mostly found in animal products, fatty meats, cheese, butter and lard. They can be extremely harmful to your health when consumed in large amounts because they clog up your arteries. They are best consumed in moderation.

You should never touch trans fats. Trans fatty acids (trans fats) aren't usually found in nature. Scientists manufacture them in a lab to ensure a longer shelf life for packaged foods. They are often found in fried foods, chips, French fries, crackers, corn chips, cakes and many other items, and they are extremely harmful to your body on a cellular level.

Let me explain. All of your individual cells are coated in fat known as a lipid bi-layer. This coating acts as the brain of the cell. (I, like many doctors, used to think the nucleus was the brain. But it has been recently discovered that the cell can survive without the nucleus, but not the lipid bi-layer.)

That being said, your body will use any fat available—including trans fats—to build cell walls. The problem with using trans fats to do this is that because they are unnatural, they have a different shape than naturally occurring fats. Trans fats are shaped like Z's and normal fats are shaped like C's, meaning that they don't fit together when layered. This makes for a very weak cell wall. Weak cell walls make for weak cells, and therefore weak systems and organs. Much like simple sugars, everyone should stay away from these fats at all costs. They do you no good. They were developed by scientists in the lab to make your food last longer than you. That is not normal or healthy to eat.

The Power of Proteins

You have tens of thousands of different proteins that act as the building blocks of your cells. The variety and specialization of these proteins is far ranging, but all of them are made up of the same 25 basic amino acids. Your body produces some of these on its own, but many of them you must consume.

If you are deficient in amino acids, it's going to manifest itself in numerous symptoms, including weight gain. However, one of the primary symptoms is decreased brain function. Your brain uses protein to communicate with the rest of your body, so a deficiency will cause mood problems, anxiety, depression, stress and sleep disorders. It's also well known that protein is the building block for muscle development, which is crucial for weight management.

Essential amino acids are proteins your body cannot make, therefore you must get them through your diet. They include histidine, isoleucine, leucine, lysine, methionine, phenylalanine, threonine, tryptophan and valine.

Non-essential amino acids are produced by your body when everything is functioning on an optimal level. They include alanine, arginine, aspartic acid, cysteine, glutamic acid, glutamine, glycine, proline, serine, tyrosine, asparagine and selenocysteine.

Conditional amino acids are typically made by your body, but some people need to supplement the production of these amino acids based on different lifestyle choices or illnesses. They include cysteine, cystine, glutamine, taurine and tyrosine.

2. What are Micronutrients?

These tiny vitamins and minerals make up a small part of your diet, but the impact they have on your health is huge. Without them your body's vital organs cannot perform optimally. In functional medicine, those listed below are the key vitamins and minerals we look for.

Vitamin A

Aids in immune function, skin and bone growth, vision and mucus formation. Different forms of vitamin A are found in various animal and plant food sources. Some of the top vitamin A-containing foods include carrots, dark leafy greens, and chicken and beef liver.

Vitamin B Complex

There are 11 different vitamins belonging to the vitamin B complex, and all of them are crucial to creating or maintaining optimal health and weight. These vitamins help with brain function, thyroid function, sleep patterns and metabolism. Deficiencies show up as fatigue, poor memory, irritability and gastrointestinal disturbances.

Vitamin C

Cannot be stored in your body and must be consumed from your diet. It is important for stress and cortisol management and helps with immune system health by combating free radical damage to your cells. It also helps lower blood pressure.

Vitamin D

Actually a hormone produced naturally in your body when exposed to the sun. But because you can also consume it through food, many people rely on their diet for their daily doses. Vitamin D is crucial for bone and teeth development, aids in thyroid and insulin production and calcium absorption. Lack of this vitamin has been connected to osteoporosis, muscle spasms, autoimmune diseases, depression, migraines, polycystic ovary syndrome and almost every chronic disease known. Low levels of vitamin D are associated with cancer, disease and obesity.

Vitamin E

An antioxidant found in many nuts, seeds and oils. Vitamin E is very effective at soothing inflammation and lowering cholesterol. A deficiency in this vitamin has been linked to heart disease, PMS, fibrocystic breast disease and restless leg syndrome.

Vitamin K

Found in egg yolks and green leafy vegetables, this vitamin helps in collagen production, bone growth, blood clotting, calcium management and more.

Calcium

You have more calcium in your body than any other mineral, and it makes up the majority of your bones and teeth. It is also necessary for hormone regulation and energy production. If you are defi t in calcium you are susceptible to high blood pressure, muscle spasms and osteoporosis. Cheeses and dark green vegetables are good sources of calcium.

Copper

A mineral used to maintain the health of many of your vital organs, including your heart, brain, kidneys and liver. It is responsible for metabolizing many other vitamins and minerals, regulating immune function and hormone production. Anemia, fatigue and suppressed immune function are all symptoms of low copper intake.

Magnesium

Important for two major biological functions: energy production and bone loss prevention. It also aids in nerve function, sleep patterns and immune system function. A deficiency in magnesium can result in fatigue, depression, anxiety, muscle spasms, fibromyalgia, constipation, migraine headaches and insomnia.

Potassium

An electrolyte that is essential for muscle and nerve function. If you are lacking in this mineral your muscles may get extremely weak or painful, and you might experience heart problems and nervous system failure.

Zinc

Although you only need a small amount of it, zinc plays a very important role in your body. It is hugely important for hormone production, immune efficiency and bone and skin health.

WHAT DOES MALNUTRITION LOOK LIKE? COMPREHENSIVE CHECK FOR GASTROINTESTINAL HEALTH*

- Irritable bowel syndrome (IBS)
- Less than one bowel movement daily
- Straining, hard stools or incomplete emptying
- Abdominal discomfort, bloating, distention or excess gas
- Bowel symptoms that resolve with defecation
- Change in frequency or appearance of stool
- Nausea
- Heartburn, indigestion or GERD
- Stomach ulcers or gastritis
- Loose or unformed stools
- Colitis or diverticulitis
- Recurrent yeast infections
- Sugar cravings
- Drink alcohol more than once weekly
- Antibiotic usage in the past two years
- Chronic sinus congestion
- Foggy or daytime sleepiness
- Anemia
- B 12 or other vitamin deficiency
- Pet owner
- Travel or living abroad

*DISCLAIMER: The Cracking the Bikini Code program may help alleviate many of the symptoms described above, but it is in no way intended to replace medical treatment from a physician. In addition, those who are suffering from advanced diabetes, renal failure or are undergoing treatment for cancer should absolutely not attempt this program. You should always consult with your doctor about whether this, or any similar program is appropriate for you and how your current medications could be affected by a weight loss program of this nature.

HOW THE BIKINI CODE ADDRESSES MALNUTRITION

Revamping your diet is a large part of the program, but that alone will not get you off the road to malnutrition, although it's a good start. Eating foods that supply your body with the nutrients I mentioned in this chapter is crucial to slimming down and getting healthy. (As I have mentioned, I have provided a day-to-day diet plan in Part III of this book.)

However, the issue becomes more complicated because even those who think they eat healthy and get plenty of nutrition still often lack many vital vitamins and minerals. This is because in this day and age you can't eat your way to optimal nutrition. Over-farming and processing practices have left many of our foods nutritionally depleted.

That is why all-natural supplementation is also a major component to the program. Functional medicine relies on high-quality nutritional supplementation. These supplements are much different from your average daily multi-vitamins and are regulated for purity and potency by functional medicine standards. I have found that 100 percent of my patients are in need and can benefit form oral supplementation.

In severe cases where patients are experiencing extreme deficiencies, intravenous (IV) nutritional therapies (which must be administered in-office by a functional medicine practitioner) can greatly expedite the process of replenishing your body of missing nutrients.

That said, the major three nutritional tools functional medicine uses to heal patients are diet, supplementation and IV nutritional therapies.

BIKINI CODE BOTTOM LINE

You may be surprised to learn that malnutrition is a common occurrence in modern-day Americans. But functional medicine has proved that not all foods are created equal, and that proper nutrition is like the wheels of a car. You are not going to get very far if you don't have them. This is why **Key No. 5 to Cracking the Bikini Code is to Nutrify Your Body Properly.**

HOW FRAN CRACKED THE BIKINI CODE

Because she was overweight, no one would have guessed that when Fran first walked into my office at 39 years old many of her symptoms and problems were related to severe malnutrition. Her list of ailments was extensive and included intense chronic aches and pains (fibromyalgia), sleep apnea and depression. She had been to many mainstream doctors who gave her a bevy of pain medications, anti-depressants, sleeping pills and apparatuses, none of which ever gave her long-term relief. Her pain kept her from trying any sort of exercise, which also contributed to the 89 pounds of excess weight she was battling.

She admitted to me that she was afraid to try another doctor and was reluctant to tell me what was wrong because she thought I, like all the other doctors, would simply say they couldn't find anything really wrong with her and that it was all in her head. Many of her family members also had negative reactions to her complaints and insistence that something was really wrong, and she had become very isolated from her loved ones. She was petrified of living a lonely, miserable existence forever.

Fran was right though. There was something very wrong with her. The tests revealed that she was severely deficient in vitamin D, selenium, magnesium, and amino acids, which are the building blocks of everything in the body. She also had cortisol problems and suffered from overall slightly decreased thyroid levels.

Once I realized how many nutrients she was lacking, it was clear why she was in so much pain. So my job became cleaning out all the bad food and then nutrifying her. In Phase I, I put her on the Bikini Code diet and she lost 23 pounds and began the detoxifying process. She immediately started noticing improvement in her pain issues, but it was in Phase II when I placed her on IV nutrient therapies that things really started to improve. After the first six sessions she noticed immediate benefits, most notably bursts of energy that lasted a few days and markedly less pain. Those periods of time lasted longer and longer with each session and eventually her pain levels got so low she was able to start exercising. She continued to lose another 40 pounds and her fibromyalgia became nonexistent. Her relationships with her friends and family have improved drastically because she no longer complains. Instead, she preaches about the importance of nutrition. She said she feels like she has a whole new lease on life.

Tips for Success
[NUTRIFY YOUR BODY]

1. Remember you don't have to be starving—or even thin—to be undernourished. Excess fat does not equal excess nutrition.

2. Do take a broad-based multivitamin, mineral and nutrient supplement daily; however, be fanatical about the quality. Most regular daily types won't put a dent in your nutritional issues.

3. Don't listen to supplement fads. They can cause worse imbalances if taken incorrectly.

4. Understand that your diet and high-grade supplements are the best way to fuel your body for optimal health.

5. If upon testing your vitamin and mineral deficiencies are found to be significant enough to warrant IV nutrient therapy know that you will likely not get rid of your symptoms without it.

CHAPTER 6

Instill Awareness of Your Mental, Emotional and Spiritual Health

"I rock a bikini all summer long. I know that it's not normal, but I just don't care. I live once."

— Liz Phair, singer, songwriter

AT THIS POINT YOU SHOULD HAVE A GOOD IDEA OF HOW hormones, toxicity and malnutrition all affect your weight and health. With this knowledge, you are well on your way to your own bikini body. But there is one more key. And it is a big one. **Key No. 6 to Cracking the Bikini Code is to Instill an Awareness of Your Mental, Emotional and Spiritual Health**.

This is often the hardest one for my patients to get, and one that mainstream medicine largely ignores altogether. But I promise you without a healthy state of mind you will never achieve optimal health or weight.

The greatest example I have of how mental, emotional and spiritual health affect physical health comes from an early functional medicine patient of mine named Mary. Mary was a 50-year-old mother of three children, who worked part time. She had all the classic symptoms of hormone imbalance, toxicity and malnutrition, including extra weight, fatigue and irritability. Like many patients who are mothers, she said she didn't care for herself properly because she put everyone else's needs in front of her own. She was now seeing the consequences.

Desperate to feel better, she signed up for my program (which you are about to learn all about in the next chapter) and did very well. In three months, she lost over 30 pounds and saw a huge relief from many of her symptoms. She had increased energy, her aches and pains went away and she was sleeping eight hours a night. For many months, Mary continued to lose weight and go down the path toward optimal health. It seemed as if she had changed her life forever.

Then, one day she showed up in my office, and I couldn't believe what I saw. She had obviously gone back to her old habits. She had gained back all the weight and more. The fatigue, aches and pains were creeping back into her body. I was flabbergasted. She had been so receptive to the program and went to great lengths to understand the science behind why functional medicine works. How could she be back to this?

When I sat down and talked to Mary she explained that she had indeed stopped doing the program and courageously admitted she needed help. At first I didn't know what to do. She knew better than most that if she nourished herself properly and removed all the toxic items from her life, then her body functioned on a much higher level. She had seen the proof for herself. So I started to ask questions about the likely cause of her backslide—her mental, emotional and spiritual state.

For almost an hour, we talked about what was going on with her thoughts, feelings, beliefs, attitudes and actions. We talked and talked and eventually we came to understand that on some level she was sabotaging herself and her health. Why would she do that?

As we explored, I came to understand that there was a lot of negativity in her life. She admitted that she often had thoughts about not performing well enough at her job, or that she was a bad mother for not spending enough time with her three young children. She was very hard on herself, and so she was always in a very negative place.

But her struggles went even deeper than that. When we really started to look at her attitudes, beliefs and actions, we started to get at the root. As she started telling me more about her life, she told me one of her biggest regrets in life was that she never went to college. She grew up in a family that didn't value women's education, and so her creativity and dreams of becoming a biologist were thwarted from the time she was a child. Adding to the dysfunction, her father was an alcoholic, and so she became an emotional caretaker of sorts for the family.

Because of this, she learned to completely neglect herself. So much so, Mary admitted that caring for herself felt like betraying the ones she loved. This also led her to hold the belief that she was not worthy of being cared for the way she cared for others, or having a beautiful body and good health. She felt it was her lot in life to be stuck with an overweight, failing and aging body that didn't serve her well or look appealing.

We also learned as we talked that the only way she knew how to deal with all that negativity was with food. And that's what eventually took her over again. It was a mental, emotional and spiritual breakthrough in and of itself, but the real shocker came at the end of our talk.

As we started making all sorts of connections between her physical health and mental, emotional and spiritual health, other light bulbs started going off. She realized that not only did her parents not support her, but her current spouse also didn't support her. Then the big discovery came. She said on some level being unattractive physically gave her an excuse to not be sexual with her husband, whom she deeply, secretly resented. "A convenient barrier" is what she called it.

MORE COMMON THAN NOT

I was very glad that Mary and I were able to figure out the real reason why she felt it was necessary to remain unhealthy and unattractive. But all of this got me thinking about some of my other patients who were struggling with the program.

I have found that after most people get all the information in the program they say: "Great, this all makes sense, I'm going to do it." But invariably, everyone falls into one of two groups. The first group takes the information and is well on their way. They eat the right foods, take their supplements and change their weight and lives forever. They come back with bright eyes, clear skin, no aches or pains and much thinner. They are vibrant and have great enthusiasm for what they are doing for themselves.

Then, there is the other group. I call them the seventy-five-percenters. They understand all the information I give them, and believe that if they follow my advice they can change their lives. But in one area or another they fall short. Maybe they eat or drink things they know cause them great harm. Or they don't take the necessary measures to help detoxify and nutrify themselves. Or they neglect to complete one aspect of the program.

For the longest time I couldn't figure out why there were so many seventy-five-percenters. I knew they all desperately wanted to feel better, and I knew they had all the knowledge and resources, but they continued to practice harmful behaviors. But after going through that event with Mary, I realized there is most likely something mentally, spiritually or emotionally imbalanced that is keeping them attached to their unhealthy habits.

WHAT IS MENTAL, EMOTIONAL AND SPIRITUAL HEALTH?

Your mental, emotional and spiritual health is directly connected to your beliefs, attitudes and actions. It deals with how you see yourself, others and the world around you. When these things are in a negative or unhealthy state it creates stress in your body, which as you know greatly impacts your weight and health. In other words, negative emotions are another stress factor you need to address in order to get your bikini body and optimal health.

Mental Health

It's hard to really separate the three different categories because they are all very integrated. But the best way I can explain the mental portion is that it encompasses your thoughts and knowledge about what is happening or has happened in your life.

For example, let's say your cat jumped onto a table and knocked over an antique vase that belonged to your great-grandmother. Those are the facts. Your ability to process what happened accurately is a sign of how your mental faculties are working. Problems in this area include memory loss, difficulty paying attention, cognitive problems or a general sense of dulling of the mind.

Emotional Health

Emotional health is how you feel about the mental facts that you have. It is a reaction to the facts; and those reactions are determined by what you believe about yourself, your world and the things in it.

If you chose to get upset about your great-grandmother's vase being broken, it means that you believe it to be valuable. In order to do that, you have to first place value on the vase. No one else can. Nothing is in itself good or bad; it only has the meaning you assign to it. This means you create the belief that it should make you upset if it is broken. I believe that all meaning in your environment is assigned and consciously decided. Your culture, upbringing and surroundings all influence your reactions, but once you are aware of them you can change and control them yourself.

Spiritual Health

Spiritual health is a belief in something greater than yourself, and a belief in the ultimate oneness of all of us. Having a healthy recognition of the idea that there is something greater than yourself is extremely important in helping you connect with and appreciate the world around you.

This connection does not have to be based on a specific religion or god (although it can be). It can be as simple as recognizing that whatever force created the sun, the stars and the ocean also created you. A detachment from this connection often results in self-sabotaging habits similar to Mary's.

A part of recognizing this belief is to understand that some things are out of your control, but are all part of something larger. So instead of getting upset about the vase, maybe you think about some artist using the shards to make a piece of art, keeping your great-grandmother's spirit alive. Or maybe you will meet a new friend while shopping for a piece of décor to replace the vase. When you have this type of trust with the universe, then you are able to work through stress peacefully.

WHAT DOES A MENTAL, EMOTIONAL AND SPIRITUAL IMBALANCE LOOK LIKE?

COMPREHENSIVE CHECK OF MENTAL, EMOTIONAL AND SPIRITUAL HEALTH*

Mental
- Poor memory
- Lack of creativity
- Difficulty concentrating
- General dullness of the mind
- Cognitive dysfunction

Emotional
- Depression
- Anxiety, fear
- Frequent irritability
- Anger problems
- Unstable emotions

Spiritual
- Low self-esteem
- Overall negative outlook on life
- Low drive for life
- Inability to see good things in your life
- Lack of respect for yourself or others

*DISCLAIMER: The Cracking the Bikini Code program may help alleviate many of the symptoms described above, but it is in no way intended to replace medical treatment from a physician. In addition, those who are suffering from advanced diabetes, renal failure or are undergoing treatment for cancer should absolutely not attempt this program. You should always consult with your doctor about whether this, or any similar program is appropriate for you and how your current medications could be affected by a weight loss program of this nature.

HOW THE BIKINI CODE PROGRAM ADDRESSES
A MENTAL, EMOTIONAL AND SPIRITUAL IMBALANCE

One of the key ways that I help patients with a mental, emotional and spiritual imbalance is by teaching them how to elicit a natural relaxation response in their own body. The relaxation response is a physiological process that evolved to calm your nervous system after a stressful situation. Most animals in the wild have a version of this process.

For modern people who have undergone large amounts of chronic stress (internal or external), figuring out how to capture and use this response is important to getting your cortisol balanced. And, if you have your emotions under control, you can prevent all sorts of damaging habits that are keeping you from optimal health. These damaging habits might include binge eating or drinking, addictive behavior, angry outbursts, anxious patterns and depressive thoughts.

The best way to elicit this relaxation response in people is through introspective activities such as meditation, prayer and journaling. All of these activities encourage your brain to release chemicals that quiet your nervous system, resetting your emotions.

BIKINI BODY BOTTOM LINE

You may discount the impact your mental, emotional and spiritual health has on your physical health, but that would be a huge mistake. If you fail to address this aspect of your life and wellbeing, you will probably not get where you want to be and lose weight. Successfully addressing this component with the appropriate tools will ensure that you accomplish your health and weight goals.

HOW ANNE BECAME TRULY BALANCED

Anne was in her mid-30s and about 25 pounds overweight when she made her first appointment with me. Her chief complaint was that she felt depressed. This became very obvious when I simply asked her what she was sad about, and she was immediately on the verge of crying. When she was finally able to open up it was like releasing a flood- gate. She said she was not really happy with work (she owned her own business) and felt trapped because she no longer wanted to run it. She also struggled with her personal relationships and said she and her husband had not had sex in years. It was so bad they didn't even talk about it and had essentially resolved to just be like friends, sleeping in separate beds. She had very few friends and no outside hobbies because work consumed most of her time.

This was especially hard for her because she had always wanted to be an artist and had a talent for pottery. In fact, when she was younger she was accepted to a specialized arts school but her parents wouldn't let her go because they wanted her to do something practical. It didn't take long to realize a lot of her stress and health problems actually had to do with her inability to express her creativity.

What I found after putting her through the tests was that she also had high blood pressure, yeast overgrowth, imbalanced cortisol and nutritional deficiencies. I started her on supplements, but despite that correction and multiple attempts, she failed. It was obvious to me she needed mental, emotional and spiritual help first before she could fix these other problems.

Although she had all the tools in the program to help her symptoms, she found that she repeatedly sabotaged herself, eating things that were not in her best interest, skipping supplements, switching high-quality supplements for cheaper drug store versions that appeared to be equal but were not. She always had excuses for not exercising and never grasped the importance of integrating relaxation response exercises into her life. After struggling for a long time, she soon realized if she didn't get her head right, she would never get her body right.

Eventually, she used the Cracking the Bikini Code workbook to discover that not fulfilling her love of art had left her frustrated and stressed. The stress caused by this was creating a severe hormone imbalance, which resulted in depression. Once she realized what was actually at the core of her problems, she knew what she had to do. She had a discussion with her husband, and they figured out a way for her to be able to quit the business and pursue her passion. The results of this conversation and the subsequent life changes were astounding. She not only instantly felt happier and less stressed, but also talking through their emotions and setting new goals, brought them closer again. They were able to rekindle their marriage, and even start sleeping in the same bed again.

Tips for Success

1. Spend time evaluating your thoughts, feelings, beliefs and actions. They have a much greater impact on your physical health than you might suspect.

2. An easy way to begin that process is to start journaling. It allows you to notice what you are noticing and explore what you learn about yourself.

3. Try to identify your underlying beliefs as they ultimately determine your thoughts, feelings and actions.

4. Talking with someone else can help you clarify what you feel.

Don't underestimate the importance of this. It is no different from missing a leg. If you don't address it, it is going to make it really hard to walk. If you don't get your head right, you will never get your body right. So, let's do the work.

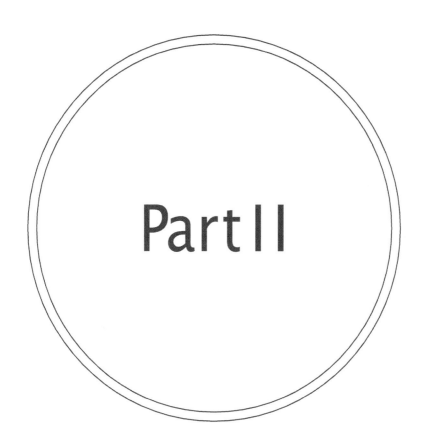

Part II

CHAPTER 7

The Bikini Code Program

"Women shop for a bikini with more care than they do a husband. The rules are the same. Look for something you'll feel comfortable wearing. Allow for room to grow."

— Erma Bombeck, writer, humorist

NOW YOU HAVE ALL THE SECRETS TO WEIGHT LOSS success. The 6 Keys to Cracking the Bikini Code contain all the information you need to know to transform your body and life. Let's briefly review them.

B - Be Honest About Your Health

Listen to what your body is saying. Don't just cover up symptoms—which includes extra weight. Get at the root of your health problems.

I - Inform Yourself

Don't settle for the standard of care recognized by mainstream medicine. Realize you do have other options, and seek out more natural remedies when possible.

K - Keep Your Hormones Balanced

Hormones govern almost every function in your body Keeping them balanced is essential when addressing weight loss and many other symptoms that plague you.

I - Illuminate and Eliminate Toxins In Your Body

Our modern world and our bodies are filled with toxic chemicals. The ability to recognize and rid your life of these toxins is crucial to optimal health and weight loss.

N - Nutrify Your Body

Understand the power of a clean diet and proper nutritional supplementation. Giving your cells high quality fuel allows them to function on an optimal level.

I - Instill an Awareness of Mental, Emotional & Spiritual Health

Your health is a direct product of your mental state. Your weight and body will never be truly optimal if you don't address your mind and life—they are all intertwined.

THE BIKINI CODE PROGRAM

Got it? Great. Now, it is time to put these keys into action. The Cracking the Bikini Code program is broken down into three phases. For each phase, I will give you specific instruction on how to balance your hormones, nutrition, toxicity levels, and mental, emotional and spiritual health.

Phase I is a six-week rapid weight loss and detoxification phase, in which you will loose a significant amount of weight (about 20 to 30 pounds) and begin to detoxify your body.

Phase II is a three-month program designed to begin healing all of your biological systems and continue your weight loss progress. This is where the majority of patients actually lose the most weight.

And Phase III is the ongoing portion. It is all about tweaking and customizing a program that you can sustain on a long-term basis.

In the following chapters, I will give you directions for navigating these phases, but first I want to give you an overview of what you can expect in each phase.

Bikini Code Tests

This is where the process gets really interesting. All of the recommended functional medicine tests are cutting-edge and scientifically advanced to detect exactly how your individual cells and organ systems are performing. With these tests, I guarantee you will learn more about your body, your weight and your symptoms than you ever thought possible.

Each phase has a unique set of tests. In the next three chapters you will learn about each test in detail. Right now, just know that all of these tests are designed to get at the core of your weight and health issues and never mask them. Each test is chosen based on sensitivity and specificity.

And while we are on the subject of testing, it is important to reiterate that functional medicine uses higher standards for reading test results than you're used to with your regular doctor. Our goal is to get you off the road to diabetes, cancer, heart disease or obesity, before it becomes an issue. Using higher standards, we look for optimal function, not just absence of disease. Therefore we do not use the "normal" or "reference" values that most labs use to determine if treatment is needed or not. We use much stricter values.

The main reason for using different values is that mainstream medicine says "normal" is what pertains to 95 percent of the population. But the problem is that about 60 percent of that population is obese or overweight. As I said earlier, I don't know about you, but I don't want to be compared to a population that is saturated with health problems. I want to be compared to optimal levels of health, which is what functional medicine does.

Bikini Code Nutrition Plan

The nutrition portion of the program is hugely important. Let me say that again. It is crucial to your success. As I've said before, failing to address this aspect is like not putting tires on your car. Where do you think you're going without the tires on your car?

Like the tests, each phase has a different diet plan. The first phase includes an easy-to-follow detoxification diet that works for most everyone. The second and third phases include nutritional plans that can be completely customized to address your specific nutritional and health needs.

All of the phases will teach you how to eat fresh, non-toxic foods on a daily basis and ditch all those nasty chemicals and harmful foods that are keeping you fat and sick. I've included many recipes to make things as easy and delicious as possible for you.

Bikini Code Supplements

Another point I hit home time and time again: You can't eat your way to complete nutrition in this day and age. And it's true. No matter how many avocados, pomegranates or other "superfoods" you eat, you will still need some additional support. As I said earlier, the main reason for this is because in this country the farmlands have been overworked and food has been mass-produced and processed for decades. Many foods are deficient in nutrients because of this. But also, because your body has been neglected for so long, you are going to need high doses of supplements in order to get you back to where you should be.

In addition, supplements provide a natural way of aiding in detoxification and hormone regulation that you would not normally get through your diet. This is why each phase comes with a set of supplement recommendations.

It is important to note that functional medicine supplements have a significantly greater quality, purity and potency. To give you an example, typically vitamin D is sold in 400 IU capsules, where as the one I recommend has 5,000 IUs. When taken in the right concentration, vitamins and minerals are powerful healing tools. Like everything else, the supplements I recommend vary according to the phase.

Bikini Code Exercise Plan

The requirements for physical exercise vary from phase to phase, but you can be sure that getting your body moving is an integral part of getting healthy. An exercise regimen is not included in Phase I, so you are off the hook there, but it is an extremely integral part of Phase II and III as well as lifelong achievement and maintenance of optimal health.

Bikini Code Mental, Emotional and Spiritual Plan

Because your mental, emotional and spiritual health is just as important to your bikini body as your hormones, nutrition and ability to detoxify, every phase has tools to help you balance your emotions. Those tools include access to weekly motivational emails, weekly teleclasses in which you will be able to ask questions directly, and a workbook to help you engage in self- awareness exercises, meditation and journaling. (Visit thebikinicode.com for more information.)

Bikini Body Bottom Line

Changing habits that you have been developing your entire life is going to be tough. There's no getting around it. But, I promise you that the program will give you as much guidance and support as you need to successfully complete it. With explicit guidance detailing the tools of the Bikini Code—everything from the foods you should eat, to your exercise, to stress management— if you truly want a bikini body and follow these steps, you will not fail.

Tips for Success

1. Make a commitment to yourself.

Write down all the reasons why you want to complete this program, and read them as often as you need. I encourage patients to hang up this list somewhere visible or keep it with them in a purse or wallet.

2. Visualize your bikini body.

A great way to keep your motivation high is to cut out a picture of your dream body and put a picture of your face on it. Again, put this picture somewhere you will see it on a regular basis.

3. Get your family members on board.

If you explain to your family and friends what you are doing and why, they are more likely to help you out along the way. Once they see how fantastic you feel and look, they might even want to do it with you.

4. Have patience with yourself.

Any time you start a new regimen, it is going to need some adjusting. This clean way of living and eating is not always easy, but the results will speak for themselves.

CHAPTER 8
Cleanse Your Body for Rapid Weight Loss and Detoxification: Phase 1

"It feels like I could go outside with a bikini thong on right now."

— Puff Daddy, musician, entrepreneur

THE OTHER DAY A FRIEND AND MENTOR REMINDED ME of the true power of the word "decision." She was talking about how the root of the word comes from Latin and means to cut away from (literally to de-cise). Meaning, every time you make a decision you are cutting away all your other options. When I heard this, the word instantly became more powerful to me because I realized my decisions alone could cut out the bad things in my life. You have that power, too.

Phase I is geared toward harnessing that power and deciding to cut away everything that is keeping you unhealthy and unhappy. For this phase, I designed a comprehensive, step-by-step plan to help you eliminate the things in your life that are causing hormone, toxicity, nutritional, mental, emotional and spiritual imbalances.

As a result of addressing these things, you can expect to lose about 20 and 30 pounds of fat in six weeks. You will also experience a thorough detoxification for your body, preparing it for healing in Phases II and III. And your body will instantly start to thank you in all kinds of wonderful ways. Many of your other symptoms will start to subside; you will start sleeping better, your mood will elevate and you will have infinitely more energy. If all that sounds good, then let's get started!

BIKINI CODE TESTS: PHASE I

When entering into Phase I, I typically start by giving patients a functional medicine test to gauge their overall level of health. I call it my "thermometer," and it, along with an extensive patient questionnaire, helps determine exactly where someone is starting.

This test is administered by using an advanced technology called a bioelectrical impedance analysis (BIA). A BIA works by having a physician strategically place electrodes on your body that give off highly sensitive, yet harmless, electrical impulses. As the impulses travel through your body they bounce back with all kinds of information, but there are two main areas of concentration. This test should be administered in-office and under the care of a functional medicine physician. The results are immediate and will inform you about the following two items.

1. Body Composition Analysis

This reading gets straight to the fat. Because the highly sensitive waves react differently to various tissues and substances in your body, they measure exact amounts of fat, muscle and water. This gives you a clear picture of how much fat (read toxins) is in your body, if you are properly hydrated, and where you are with your muscle mass. This test is exceedingly more accurate and detailed than a typical body mass index (BMI) chart or pinchers.

2. Phase Angle

On a more microscopic level, the electrical impulses also detect the strength and resilience of your individual cell walls. This is important because when your cell walls are weak they can't perform properly. Problems here primarily indicate toxicity issues.

BIKINI CODE NUTRITION PLAN: PHASE I

The test is very informative about your starting point, but the bulk of this phase deals with revolutionizing the way you eat. This means no more toxic foods or foods that feed toxic yeasts in your gut. It's time to start thinking "fresh." To make the transition as easy as possible, I have created a step-by-step, six-week nutrition plan to foster detoxification and rapid weight loss. It starts on page 103. The plan has three purposes.

1. Low Glycemic Index

The first principle is to eat foods with a low glycemic index. As you learned in previous chapters, this is crucial to stabilizing your blood sugar, which in turn stabilizes your insulin hormones and thus the rest of your master hormones. Also, remember that a high glycemic load triggers your body to make and store fat.

2. Fresh Foods

Say good-bye to all processed foods. They are nutritionally depleted and are of no real value to your body. Additionally, they contain toxic preservatives, added flavorings and colorings. These unusable toxins not only inflame your digestive organs, but also they contribute heavily to weight gain because your body stores them in fat and other tissues. But don't worry, I promise that once you start eating fresh foods, you will never go back.

3. Fight Inflammation

Last but not least, this plan eliminates the most common gastrointestinal irritants in the modern diet. These things include: sugars, trans fats, processed foods, dairy products, alcohol, gluten and artificial flavors, colors and preservatives.

Now that you know the three principles behind the plan, let's get down to the specifics. This detox and weight loss phase gives your body an immediate and impactful sense of relief. All of your digestive organs, from your mouth to your bottom, will become happier and less inflamed. Your detoxification organs—the liver, kidneys and skin—will get a much-needed break from being overworked. And even the most highly sensitive of systems, your endocrine and nervous systems, will become significantly less stressed—all from just changing the way you eat and the supplements you take. And don't worry; this is just temporary. In the next phase, you will get to eat many more foods and calories.

Protein

Many of my patients love the fact that fresh meats are a staple of the diet. You can enjoy a variety of beef, seafood and chicken recipes; just remember they have to be fresh. Canned, cured or marinated meats often contain harmful chemicals and seasoning agents. Your goal is to eliminate processed foods from your diet during this program.

Each day, women are allowed two 3.5-ounce portions of meat (men can have two 5-ounce portions). You can eat your two servings at any two meals during the day. However, I recommend dinner as one of them because it is important to get protein before you go to sleep.

Beef and seafood are slightly limited, and you should only have two to three servings of each per week. Lean meats like chicken breasts should make up the rest of your meals.

It is important to choose high-quality meats (organic is best) because they are your best source of those all-important proteins we discussed in Chapter 5.

*Vegetarians can follow this program too; they simply need to substitute a high protein shake for the meat portions.

Vegetables

Many of the same standards apply to your vegetables. You should not eat anything processed. Everything should be fresh or frozen and organic when possible. This is extremely important in helping to detoxify your body and lose weight.

These vegetables will supply your body with vitamins, minerals, nutrients, low glycemic calories and fiber, all of which help balance your hormones, detoxify and nutrify.

Fruits

Fruits, on the other hand, are a little more limited because they naturally contain higher levels of sugar. There are a few low glycemic varieties, however, and they include green apples, grapefruits, strawberries and oranges (any type of orange is fine). Each day you can have two pieces of fruit. Note that a whole grapefruit counts for two servings of fruit though.

Snacks and Dressings

Snacking is important to keep your blood sugar stable. You can get Melba toast, Melba rounds and Grissini bread sticks (gluten free, as it is one of the most common sensitivities). They will give you a nice, satisfying crunch.

For a veggie or salad dressing, I recommend apple cider vinegar and MCT oil (which you will learn more about shortly). MCT oil is your best source of healthy fat during Phase I. Healthy fats are important for brain function, metabolism and a host of other things related to weight loss. If you are not eating a lot of salads, I encourage you to drink one tablespoon of MCT oil by itself on a daily basis.

I also suggest you consume the juice of one lemon per day. Lemon juice is a natural detoxifier as it helps clean and flush your body. You can squeeze it on vegetables, or mix it with water. It is totally up to you. This lemon juice does not count toward your fruit serving for the day.

Drinks

You can drink water, decaffeinated tea and decaffeinated coffee to your heart's content. But leave all the other drinks, including alcohol and diet drinks, alone. You must avoid caffeine because it raises cortisol levels. Also, alcohol is a toxin that directly affects your intestinal lining. It also affects your blood sugar levels and throws off your hormonal balance. Diet drinks increase sweet cravings and they contain harmful chemicals. There are more complaints to the FDA about aspartame than any other food or drug.

To sweeten your drinks you can use Stevia, Truvia or xylitol, which are the only all-natural low-calorie sweeteners allowed on this program. Avoid all other sweeteners, honey, syrups or sugars.

BIKINI CODE SUPPLEMENTS: PHASE I

Many of the Phase I supplements are geared toward infusing your system with pure, high quality vitamins and minerals, and other nutrients. The others aid in detoxification, hormone balance and appetite suppression.

During Phase I, everyone should take physician formulated pharmaceutical grade supplements that accomplish the following:

(Visit thebikinicode.com for purchasing information).

1. Metabolic Stimulators

Herbs such as African mango, rhodiola, astragalus and pygeum, along with amino acids such as carnitine, arginine, ornithine and glutamine may increase fat metabolism in the body.

2. Detoxification Support for Liver and Colon

A blend of natural herbs and vitamins, such as artichoke, watercress, milk thistle, alpha lipoic acid, n-acetyl-cysteine, green tea extract, pomegranate extract, methylsulfonylmethane, calcium d-gucarate, magnesium, aloe, triphala extract or fiber will help stimulate liver and colon function.

3. Mineral Support

This should include a comprehensive formula to address a variety of common mineral deficit contributing to weight gain and that includes calcium, iodine, magnesium, zinc, selenium, copper, manganese, chromium, molybdenum, potassium malic acid and others.

4. MCT Oil
Provides your body with an essential form of energy by giving your body a source of healthy fats. These types of fats are thought to help boost your metabolism, regulate your hormones and regulate blood sugar.

5. B Vitamin Support
B vitamins are necessary for energy production in the body and for burning fat for weight loss. All B vitamins including thiamine, riboflavin, niacin, B6, folate, B12, biotin and pantothenic acid should be included.

6. Thyroid Support
A multi-glandular mineral and herbal formula to support the thyroid that includes iodine, selenium, adrenal and thyroid extracts, tyrosine, pituitary, bladderwrack, spleen and thymus will support weight loss very well.

7. Carbohydrate Craving Control
To help create balance in the brain and a feeling of wellbeing that satiates cravings, a supplement that contains nutrients such as phenylalanine, tyrosine, glutamine and hydroxytryptophan, chromium and B6 will help.

*These statements have not been evaluated by the Food and Drug Administration. These products are not intended to diagnose, treat, cure or prevent any disease.

ITEMS TO ELIMINATE DURING PHASE I

Even small things make a big difference. While foods and beverages are probably the largest contributing factor to toxicity issues, they certainly aren't the only factors. Here is a list of other items you should probably consider double-checking.

1. Toothpaste
Switch to an all-natural toothpaste brand that doesn't use fluoride or other harmful toxins. I suggest Tom's toothpaste, which comes in many different flavors.

2. Antiperspirant

Many deodorants are filled with heavy metals like aluminum, which are extremely toxic to your system and build up over time. Choosing an all-natural deodorant can help eliminate those metals from your system while keeping you feeling fresh.

3. Lotions

Use only water-based lotions or an MCT oil moisturizer. Do not use lotions with processed oils in them. Your body absorbs these fats no different than something you put in your mouth and it will prevent you from losing weight.

BIKINI CODE EXERCISE PLAN: PHASE I

This might come as a nice surprise to you: while exercise is key to maintaining long-term weight loss, during this phase you should not begin exercising. Because you are drastically changing your lifestyle, your body shouldn't endure stress at this moment.

BIKINI CODE MENTAL, EMOTION AND SPIRITUAL EXERCISE PLAN: PHASE I

But that doesn't mean you don't have to work out your brain to address the all-important mental, emotional and spiritual aspect of the program. I recommend you spend 20 minutes twice a day completing relaxation response exercises that address your mental, emotional and spiritual state.

These exercises can include meditation, restorative yoga and yogic breathing exercises known as pranayama. While you may think that you are relaxing while watching TV or going for a walk, there are certain proven chemical responses your body undergoes when participating in these relaxation response exercises that calm your nervous system and help your body recover from stressful situations. (For a list of beginner meditation tools, please see the Resource Guide on page 165)

BIKINI CODE SUPPORT SYSTEM: PHASE I

I know first-hand that drastically changing your habits can be challenging. Plus, there might be people in your life who try to talk you out of it or even call you crazy (I know there were in mine). So it is extremely important to understand that you are not in this alone. To help you power through this important detoxification phase, I've developed an online bikini body support system that you may choose to participate in.

Mental, Emotional, Spiritual Audio Files

I pre-recorded educational and inspirational audio files that correspond with the six-week program. They are made to keep you inspired and on track.

Workbook

In addition, I created a workbook that has written exercises to help you track your progress and develop emotional, mental and spiritual balance.

Forum

Also on the website, there is a forum that allows you to interact with me, my staff and other clients who are going through the program. It is great for asking questions you might have along the way.

Teleclass

As part of the program, I offer weekly teleclasses in which participants can ask questions of me and interact with other participants. Participants can easily sign up online.

(Visit thebikinicode.com for purchasing information).

BIKINI CODE BOTTOM LINE

This phase is designed to show you that you alone have the power to change your eating habits, your exercise routine, your mental state and your nutrition. All of those factors are controlled by your decisions, and all of those factors are important keys to getting your bikini body and optimal health.

This chapter hopefully makes those decisions easier by giving you a solid game plan to work with, however, none of the information matters unless you make the ultimate commitment in your mind to change your life. So, now is the time to make a commitment to completing Phase I and lose up to 30 pounds in six weeks.

TIPS FOR SUCCESS:
[CLEANSE YOUR BODY FOR RAPID WEIGHT LOSS & DETOXIFICATION]

1. Your freezer is your friend.

When you make a meal, make enough for three or four portions so you can freeze and use them for future meals. Make sure to label them clearly and include the date.

2. Plan ahead.

Get everything you need for the day (your food and supplements) prepared the night before. Better yet, cook on the weekend , and prepare enough food for the upcoming week.

3. Make it easy.

To make taking supplements easy, get some plastic bags and label them with a pen. Ration out all your supplements at one time so you don't have to think about it every day.

4. Have a plan.

Social situations can be tricky. But if you come up with a plan before you go, you will avoid temptations. For example, if I'm out with friends and there's alcohol involved, I order seltzer water with a splash of cranberry (for color) and a lime. I call it the Bikinitini.

5. Enjoy a sweet treat.

Mix together MCT oil, organic cocoa powder and Stevia. Pour it into an ice cube tray and freeze it. It's a great way to get your daily MCT oil in a tasty treat.

CHAPTER 9

Optimize Your Health with Custom Medicine: Phase II

"To look good in the water you have to pick the right swimsuit. I own close to 500."

—Amanda Beard, Olympian

A FTER COMPLETING PHASE I, YOU MOST LIKELY LOST A significant amount of weight and are starting to get relief from some of your nagging symptoms. Maybe you are sleeping better, have more energy or you notice your skin, hair and nails are healthier. These are all signs you are on the road to better health, but you are not at your destination yet. It's time to dig even deeper and feel even better.

If the theme of Phase I was all about cutting out the bad, the theme of Phase II is about digging deeper and customizing. During this phase, you will see the revolutionary way in which functional medicine determines exactly what your individual cells need. It is the opposite of one-size-fits-all medicine; it is the anti-doc-in-a-box program. Every single human body on the planet has different needs, genetic codes, stresses, compositions, lifestyles and reactions to their surrounding environment, right? So why would we all need the same drugs or multi-vitamins? The answer is we don't.

This three-month phase will pinpoint and address your specific nutritional deficiencies, food sensitivities, hormone imbalances, toxicity issues and much more. The results experienced during Phase I are dramatic. But Phase II is where you can expect to lose the most weight, find long-term solutions to your symptoms and revamp your life for good. Also, during this phase—and this is the fun part—you will learn more about your individual body than you ever thought possible.

BIKINI CODE TESTS: PHASE II

Because they are highly specialized and processed by only a handful of laboratories in the country, these test results might take longer than you are used to. That being said, if indicated, you should start these tests before you enter into Phase I so that the results are back in time for you to start Phase II on time. So what exactly are we looking for with this test information?

Hormone Test

Many mainstream doctors claim they test for hormone imbalances, but rarely do they use an accurate or complete method of testing. Often times they will make assessments based on a one-time blood sample. In functional medicine, we check your levels using numerous saliva samples from a 29-day cycle (if you are a menstruating female) or multiple times throughout one day (if you've stopped menstruating) to get a more complete picture of your hormonal cycle on different days and at different times of the day.

This test checks for testosterone, estrogen and progesterone imbalances, unhealthy cortisol levels and signs of adrenal fatigue. To round out your hormone profile, we use blood tests for thyroid and insulin problems. In the end, you will know the exact levels of your seven master hormones and where you need help. (For more information, see the Resource Guide on page 165.)

Food Sensitivity Test

This test alone is a complete game changer. A cornerstone of functional medicine, the food sensitivity test determines exactly what foods are irritating and influencing your individual gastrointestinal tract. Everyone has different food sensitivities based on his or her individual DNA and lifestyle. I have never seen anyone who didn't have some kind of issue here. Once you eliminate these foods from your system, you will see dramatic changes in many of your symptoms and problem areas.

I use the ALCAT (antigen leukocyte cellular antibody test), which is one of the most scientifically advanced food sensitivity tests available. It uses your blood to test how your body—specifically your immune system—reacts to over 350 foods, herbs and environmental products, including dyes and food coloring. Any of these irritants can cause your organ systems to become inflamed or have a reaction.

The ALCAT is far superior to any kind of skin pricking tests because it is able to detect sensitivities, not just true allergies. It has been around for over 25 years and is used for children, professional athletes and others. (For more information, see the Resource Guide on page 165.)

Gastrointestinal Health Test

It is true that you need certain bacteria inside your body to survive, but some rather shady characters can also take up residence and cause you harm. Most of these bad guys (infections) live in your gut, and as we talked about before, cause all sorts of destruction and metabolic problems. The scariest thing is you may have been living with these infections for years and not have known or written off symptoms as just gas. But the truth is these infections slowly destroy your gut. This interferes with your digestion and nutrient absorption, which is stressful to your system, so they must go.

We test for these infections of the gut using advanced stool testing methods. But it's not just all about catching the bad bugs, this test also detects inflammation, ulcerative cells, absorption issues, certain digestive diseases such as Crohn's disease and celiac, pancreatic function, immune reactions and some environmental sensitivities. There is no better indicator of what is going on with your gut. (For more information, see the Resource Guide on page 165.)

Nutrition Test

In order to track down the holes in your nutrition status, I recommend a comprehensive nutritional test that checks 165 different biochemical nutritional elements. It's a blood and urine test that looks specifically at the vitamin, mineral and nutrient content of your cells. It also reads how well your cells are using the food you eat to create energy.

We test your individual cells because functional medicine recognizes that vitamins and minerals are not just free floating in your blood. They live where they are being used—inside your cells, not outside of them.

Heart Rate Variability Test

Your heart rate is not a constant speed like a metronome. A healthy heart rate variability (HRV) reading has a huge variation in it. An unhealthy one is very monotonous. In addition, a healthy HRV recovers quickly from a stressor (like going from laying down to standing up or exercising). These readings are indicators of how your heart and nervous system react to and handle stress. Several studies have now suggested a link between negative emotions (such as anxiety and hostility) and reduced HRV. (For more information, see the Resource Guide on page 165.)

BIKINI CODE NUTRITION PLAN: PHASE II

You will be happy to know that during Phase II you are allowed to eat significantly more food than you were during Phase I. But that doesn't mean you can return to eating like you used to. Calories are limited to 1200 daily.

The Phase II nutrition plan is based largely on the results from your ALCAT (food sensitivity test). While you can now have more varieties of foods, you are only to eat foods approved on your results. You will eventually get some of the problem foods back, but you have to give your gut time to heal first. That also means still no alcohol or caffeine.

In addition, you should also adhere to the low glycemic requirements because if you haven't gotten it by now, sugar affects your cortisol and therefore your weight. So for this phase, I recommended everyone continues to say no to sugars and simple carbohydrates.

The last major part of this diet is rotation. You will most likely notice when you get your ALCAT results back that many foods you ate on a daily basis were irritating your gut. That is because our systems are built for seasonal eating. This means you must rotate your foods regularly in order to prevent your body from rejecting certain foods. The ALCAT results come with a customized rotation eating chart to help you do this correctly. I have also provided a recipe guide for this phase. However, you will need to modify the recipes to work with your personal ALCAT results.

BIKINI CODE SUPPLEMENTS: PHASE II

To optimize your health during this phase, you should take a customized combination of supplements based on your individual results from the tests I just mentioned. If you are able to do this, please see page 165 for the Resource Guide for functional medicine organizations that can assist you in finding a practitioner who knows how to read the results of these tests.

If you want the benefits of Phase II, but for some reason are unable to complete the tests or find a functional medicine physician that works for your lifestyle, you can still drastically improve your health and life with the Phase II program. I developed a program based on what the vast majority of people with excess weight need. Here are the supplement components you will need for a successful program:

(Visit thebikinicode.com for purchasing information).

1. Daily Multivitamin Mineral and Nutritional Supplement

This is a comprehensive vitamin, mineral, nutrient and herbal supplement to address the unique nutritional requirements for weight loss. Ideally, the supplement will also include essential fatty acids, CoQ10, which supports cellular energy production, and other nutrients necessary for optimal cellular function and calorie burning. This is not a one-a-day vitamin. To get everything you need, you will be taking 10 to 14 capsules of vitamins a day.

2. Adrenal Support

This includes DHEA and herbs such as ashwagandha, rhodiola and ginseng, all of which support your body's ability to respond to stress. In addition, adrenal gland extracts will help adrenals to heal and improve cortisol balance and energy.

3. Digestive Support, Healing and Repair

This is a supplement to heal the gut lining, remove toxins, inoculate with good bacteria, and nourish and support that flora as well as improve digestive capabilities for optimal nutritional function.

4. Detoxification Support

This supplement is a blend of natural herbs and vitamins, such as artichoke leaf extract, broccoli seed extract, milk thistle, goldenseal root, beet powder, and more that may help stimulate liver function and other detoxification organs and organ systems in your body.

5. Amino Acid Protein Supplementation

This supplement contains plant-based proteins that provide a well-balanced amino acid profile, which provides the building blocks for most structural and functional components in the body for optimal weight loss, health and functioning.

*These statements have not been evaluated by the Food and Drug Administration. These products are not intended to diagnose, treat, cure or prevent any disease.

BIKINI CODE PHYSICAL EXERCISE PLAN: PHASE II

Now is the time in which you should start implementing exercise into your daily routine. If you are new to exercising, then please start slow with activities such as walking for 30 minutes or taking a beginner's yoga class. Eventually, you want to build up to five or six days of exercise, incorporating both cardiovascular exercises and strength training. Ultimately, high intensity interval training (HITT) is best for weight loss. Adding resistance (weight) training twice weekly will significantly improve weight loss as well.

BIKINI CODE MENTAL, EMOTIONAL AND SPIRITUAL EXERCISE PLAN: PHASE II

It is just as important to maintain your mental exercises, too. This means maintaining the 15 to 20 minutes a day of meditating, journaling or praying. This is crucial to keeping your mental, emotional and spiritual health on the right track. In Chapter 11, you will learn much more about other things you can do to help this aspect of health.

BIKINI CODE SUPPORT SYSTEM: PHASE II

Phase II is not only about losing more weight and transforming your body into its healthiest state, but also about training you in the skills you will need to maintain this level of fitness for a lifetime.

Forum Similar to Phase 1
You have access to a forum that allows you to interact with me, my staff and other clients who are going through the program. It is great for asking questions you might have along the way.

Teleclass in Phase II
I also continue to offer weekly teleclasses giving crucial knowledge, tools and support to understand why and how to take action and give you the support you need to make these crucial changes in your life and lose the weight once and for all (For more information, see the Resource Guide on page 165.

BIKINI CODE BOTTOM LINE

In Phase I, you began addressing the Bikini Code Spiral of Stress with one-size-fits-all tools designed to help you with hormone, toxicity, nutritional, mental, emotional and spiritual imbalances. In Phase II, you will dig much deeper to better understand why these imbalances are occurring and learn how to resolve them.

TIPS FOR SUCCES
[OPTIMIZE YOUR HEALTH WITH A PLAN]

1. Take it one day at a time.

Don't let feeling overwhelmed stop you from doing what you can. Learning a new way of eating and living takes time. If you feel overwhelmed, take a few minutes to meditate about your goals and revisit the vision of your dream life.

2. Don't leave out any part of the program.

You will not get the results you are hoping for if you ignore any part of the program, especially the mental, emotional and spiritual component.

3. Don't buckle under peer pressure.

If you know you are going to be in social situations that involve eating out at a restaurant, think ahead and have a few options in your mind of what you can have. Things like steamed veggies and grilled meats.

4. Don't cheat when traveling.

Many of my patients travel for their jobs or for pleasure, and they often ask how to do the program on the road. My answer is always pack your own food and bring your supplements. It may take some planning ahead, but you will feel—and look better—because of it.

CHAPTER 10
Do It Forever: Phase III

"I just want to get married in a bathing suit. Deal with it."

— Kate Upton, model, actress

AS I MENTIONED IN THE BEGINNING OF THIS BOOK, I WAS overweight on and off throughout my whole life. After going through the first two phases of the Bikini Code program, reaching 150 pounds was an ecstatic experience for me. And boy did I savor it. I started taking my time shopping for clothes. I became much more social and began traveling to new places. Best of all, I started to enjoy cooking and eating more than ever, mainly because there was no guilt associated with it. I knew that delicious, fresh foods were serving my body and mind.

For about a year I stayed at that 150 pounds. I kept eating according to my sensitivities and nutritional needs, and kept taking the supplements. And I continued to feel great. But having experienced such overwhelming results, I found myself wanting to go deeper and deeper into what other imbalances I might fi in my body. I wanted to keep reversing the so-called "aging process." I also knew functional medicine gave me the tools to dig deeper. That's when I started tweaking.

What do I mean by tweaking? Imagine your body as a house. In Phase I, you build a strong foundation, a clean slate. In Phase II, you construct a sturdy house, using nutrition as the primary building block. Phase III is like furnishing it—or tweaking your look. This really is the fun part, and it becomes a pleasure more than work because you are already reaping the benefits.

During the tweaking phase, you will repeat some of the Phase II tests to see where your body is in terms of hormones, toxicity and nutrition. But there are also a few additional tests to check for things like heavy metals, iodine levels and more. For me, it was during this period that I lost the last 10 pounds. This is also where I finally got to have my bikini and wear it, too.

The idea of wearing a bikini had been in my mind ever since I first started to see results with a functional medicine program. And for a long time, it was my little secret wish. I didn't tell too many people about it, but it was always on my mind, and I visualized it often. It was a white bikini, to symbolize purity, vitality and rebirth. And it was in the style of Marilyn Monroe from The Seven Year Itch. Very specific, I know. I told you I am big into the power of visualization.

The more weight I lost, the more I began to actually look for this bikini. It wasn't very easy to find something so specific, but I searched and searched. I finally found it, and coincidentally right before I went to the Dominican Republic for a wedding. I packed the suit but still was unsure whether I'd actually go through with wearing it. But I mustered up the courage and put it on. I stood in the mirror and got teary eyed. I thought, Oh, my gosh! I can actually wear a bikini! I have never worn a bikini my whole life, not even in high school. That's when I got the idea for this book. I wanted all women to have the chance to feel the way I did looking in that mirror: confident, healthy, beautiful and radiant. But back to the tweaking. Here's the plan for Phase III:

Bikini Code Tests: Phase III
Hormone Test
I recommend you recheck your thyroid, insulin, cortisol and sex hormone levels. At this point it's a good idea to check metabolic by-products in your urine. This test is a little different from the saliva test you did in Phase II. This test checks your hormone levels using metabolic byproducts found in your urine. The reading gauges how much your body is processing, which indicates how much you are utilizing. This test can also indicate if you are at an increased risk for breast cancer or not and how your detoxifying systems are working. . (For more information, see the Resource Guide on page 165.)

Heavy Metal Challenge Test
The majority of Americans have toxic heavy metals in their systems, mostly from environmental factors and dental work. These heavy metals reside deep in your tissues, which is why they cause so much damage. Most mainstream doctors use a blood test to check for these, but because heavy metals are not floating around in the blood the results are usually misleading. Our test is designed to draw out these heavy metals from your tissues to your urine, stool and blood. This is the most accurate way to test for the presence of metals. (For more information, see the Resource Guide on page 165.)

Gastrointestinal Health Test

If you discovered you had significant issues with yeast, bacterial overgrowth or inflammation of the gut, I suggest that you have your gut health retested with the GI Effects test. (For more information, see the Resource Guide on page 165.)

Nutrition Test

At this point you should retake the ION test, the same test from Phase II. A new reading will tell you where there are still holes in your nutrition plan and which holes have been filled. If you have significant leaky gut issues, I recommend that you also do an ALCAT retest as part of your nutrition update at some point. (For more information, see the Resource Guide on page 165.)

Cell Function Test

This test uses anabolic and catabolic by-products found in your liver to measure how much of your body is being built up and nourished versus how much is breaking down and dying. The human body is always either growing and gaining or breaking down. There is no static point. In fact, your body's cells are actually doing both at the same time. You just want your anabolic rate to be higher. (For more information, see the Resource Guide on page 165.)

BIKINI CODE NUTRITION PLAN: PHASE III

You should continue to follow your food sensitivity diet, as specified by your ALCAT results. You can begin to slowly reintroduce certain restricted foods back into your diet, but be very mindful of how they make you feel. Also make sure the foods are still fresh and not processed. If you do want to try to reintroduce foods, you should try only one food at a time and no more than one every four days.

To help you figure out which foods might be okay, you should keep a food journal and detail any and all symptoms you are feeling. Symptoms could be obvious like gastrointestinal pain, bloating, heartburn, gas, upper respiratory issues, itchy eyes, sore throat, coughs, headaches and more. Or they could be as subtle as a mood change. Also some symptoms might not show up for a few days.

Throughout this process you will learn which foods are fixed sensitivities versus transient sensitivities. If you pay really close attention, you will learn how often you can eat foods without a reaction (I can eat gluten, but only about once a month. More than that, and I get a reaction.) You will learn that foods are like people. Some you can be around every day without irritation, and others you can only see about once a month without irritation.

Maintaining a good rotation is also encouraged so that your body doesn't develop new sensitivities. That means—do not eat the same foods every day. And as always, keep your water intake high.

BIKINI CODE SUPPLEMENTS: PHASE III

For Phase III and beyond, your supplement regimen will be customized to your results and needs. There is no set kit for this phase, and you should seek the advice of a functional medicine practitioner as you continue tweaking your individual regimen.

BIKINI CODE PHYSICAL EXERCISE PLAN: PHASE III

After initiating an exercise program in Phase II, you should continue your routine in Phase III. Also, now that hopefully you have gained some strength and endurance, you should ramp up your program and incorporate as much high intensity interval training (HITT) as possible. HITT alternates between periods of high and low activity. This type of training is known to aid with weight loss and management. Resistance or weight training at least twice weekly is also recommended.

BIKINI CODE MENTAL, EMOTIONAL AND SPIRITUAL EXERCISE PLAN: PHASE III

It is just as important to maintain your mental exercises as well. This means maintaining the 15 to 20 minutes a day of meditating, journaling or praying. This is crucial to keeping your mental, emotional and spiritual health on the right track. In Chapter 11, you will learn much more about other things you can do to help this aspect of health.

SUPPORT SYSTEM

As this stage in the game, the best support is one-on-one support from a physician who can troubleshoot and tweak your individual program. However, during this phase, you can still have access to the forum and coaches at the bikini academy if you desire.

BIKINI CODE BOTTOM LINE

The best thing for me about making it to Phase III is looking back and being so grateful for my new beautiful and gratifying life, health and body. And if you make it through Phase III, you will be astonished at the person you have become. But the tricky—and wonderful—thing about Phase III is that it never really ends. Maintaining optimal health and a bikini body physique is a lifelong journey that encourages deeper and deeper levels of health as you progress. I am still in Phase III now and constantly learn new and exciting things about my body and what is going to serve it best. I encourage you to consider Phase III an ongoing way of life. And trust me, if you do you will find greater levels of health and wellness than you ever thought possible in this life.

Tips for Success
[DO IT FOREVER]

1. Knowledge, tools and support win in the end over the quick fix. Learn as much as you can. It will serve you well the rest of your life in maintaining a healthy weight and optimum health.

2. If you are having increased symptoms or increased weight revisit your program and find what you need to adjust (exercise, supplements or foods). Be honest with yourself about what you are not doing.

3. Set periodic new goals for yourself. For instance, increase muscle mass and definition this year. Set dates to hit certain milestones. Measure and celebrate when you achieve a goal or hit a milestone. It keeps the journey interesting.

4. Switch it up—variety is the spice of life. For example, eat different foods, use different exercise activities and meditation practices.

5. What is your white bikini? Set goals and reward yourself. Enlarge and rewrite your vision periodically. Every three months refresh it a little. Every year rewrite it from scratch and ask yourself, "What would I love for my life?"

CHAPTER 11
Exercise Your Connection With a Higher Calling

"For me to even be talking about bikini confidence is crazy. If you had asked me a couple of months ago, I probably would have been like, 'What are you talking about...' so it's actually huge for me to even feel okay with putting a bikini on."

— Jordin Sparks, singer, songwriter

AT THIS POINT YOU HAVE ALL THE KNOWLEDGE, TOOLS, and support you need to Crack the Bikini Code and transform your body and health for good. With the program you just read about you have the power to naturally address your hormone imbalances, toxicity issues, nutrition problems, and mental, emotional and spiritual blocks. And once you have done so, I promise you will be able to comfortably and confidently wear any bathing suit (or anything else) you wish. Plus, you will sleep better, have an abundance of vitality and energy, get off prescription medications, and enjoy a restored drive for life.

But before you embark on your journey, I have one more tool to help you. And it's the mother of all tools, a little secret weapon I saved for last. Do you remember in Chapter 1 when I asked you to visualize your dream vacation with your dream life? Well, that type of exercise is called transformative visioning, and it is extremely powerful.

Visualization is certainly not a practice I came up with by myself. For centuries, spiritual figures, business moguls and elite athletes have called upon its power to help them reach their goals. But it is a concept rarely—if ever—used in conjunction with health and weight loss plans. Having used the practice firsthand to transform my own life and health, I'd like to change that. I believe it is the perfect complement to transformative health.

WHAT IS TRANSFORMATIVE VISIONING?

Stephen Covey, bestselling author of *7 Habits of Highly Effective People*, often talks about the principle that all things are created twice, first in the mind and then in reality. For example, take something as simple as a chair. Before a chair could ever be invented, it had to be conceived of in the mind. What would it look like? What materials would you use? How high would it be?

But this principle isn't just applied to tangible objects. Your finances, career, creativity, happiness, health, and, of course, bikini body are also all created in your mind first, whether you realize it or not. Once you recognize the power of this, however, you can manifest whatever kind of life you want. You just have to start creating it, and that starts in the mind. And that's the basic principle behind transformative visioning.

HOW TO START VISIONING: RECOGNIZING YOUR DREAM

As I said before, there are many different reasons why people might choose to practice transformative visioning. But because this book is meant to help you with weight loss and health, let's start there.

The first step in using this tool (for weight loss or anything else) is to decide what you would love for your health and life. And be specific. Think about the specific dress size you want to be, a particular bikini color you like, or the exact number of pounds you want to weigh. Also include all the other characteristics about your health you want to experience. Do you want to be medication free? Maybe you want to sleep seven to eight hours every night. Or have satisfying sex with your partner? Maybe you want to feel energized in the mornings and free of chronic aches and pains.

An important part of visioning, especially in the beginning, is writing down your vision, or dream. So when you've decided on your vision, write it down with as much specificity as possible, getting as many of your senses involved. What does your new life and body feel like? How do you feel about yourself? What does it sound like? What are people saying about you? What do you eat as a thin woman? What do you see when you look in the mirror?

An important issue to remember when writing down your dream is to write it in first person, as if it's already happened. So instead of saying, "I'm going to lose 50 pounds and get into a size four." Write down, "I am a size four, and I weigh 140 pounds. I finally booked my dream vacation and am sitting in my white bikini while listening to the sound of the ocean waves and sipping fresh coconut water." When you write it down as if it has already happened, you are harnessing the power of the creative force "I am."

Another helpful hint is to write with the law of gratitude, which states whatever you are grateful for increases. So maybe you say, "I am so happy and grateful now that I rock a bikini the way I have always wanted to. I am so happy and grateful that I am medication free."

By writing your vision in this way you start to become that dream. My life coach and mentor, Mary Morrisey always says, "You can't get to your dream, you have to come from it." And that couldn't be more true. You have to start transforming into the person you want to be by doing and saying the things that person would do. By having the thoughts and actions and doing and saying the things that person would do, you are becoming that person.

ACTING OUT YOUR VISION

Now that you have decided on a vision and written it down in present tense, with detail and gratitude, it's time to start creating it. The easiest way to do this is to simply ask yourself on a regular basis: "Are my actions getting me closer to my vision?" If the answer is no, then you know you need to alter your actions. So if you're on the verge of bingeing on a few pastries because you had a bad day at work, you can think to yourself, Would I, being a 140-pound, size-four woman with health and vitality, eat three bear claws? Of course the answer is no. No healthy, thin woman eats that many bear claws at a time.

To further strengthen your ability to transform your health, it's important to continually affirm your vision by reading it to yourself or speaking it out loud. I recommend at least three times a day, especially if you find yourself faced with fear or doubt. You can also carry note cards with abbreviated visions written on them. That way if you ever get frustrated, you can instantly remind yourself of where you are headed and not stay stuck where you are.

A COMPLETE VISION

Now that you see how transformative visioning can help your journey to a bikini body, I'm going to let you in on a little secret. Visioning is a great tool that allows you to manifest all the things you want in your life, including satisfying personal relationships, financial freedom, abundant creativity and more.

And whether you realize it or not, all of those things are actually tied directly to your health. Throughout this book I have explained that weight problems are really a manifestation of other underlying imbalances. And one of those is an imbalance in life expression, or soul expression. If your creativity is stifled or your relationships are struggling, chances are you are going to be stressed and unhappy. And by now hopefully you realize that stress and unhappiness are huge contributing factors to your health problems.

I'm going to take you through a few other categories I found that can benefit greatly from transformative visioning. If you maximize all these areas, it's bound to make your health and vitality just that much stronger.

Personal Relationships

As human beings we are born social creatures, so it should come as no surprise that many of us largely define our happiness by the success of our relationships with friends, family and peers. This is why personal relationships are extremely important to a healthy mental state. Without human contact, without the nourishment of human relationships, we will become ill.

The problem is many of us settle for personal relationships based on what we think we can have versus what we would really love. We allow people into our lives who actually harm instead of help us.

So when crafting your dream life, it is important to visualize yourself participating in the types of relationships you really want. If you want a new friend, a new lover, or just a new kind of relationship with a family member or longtime peer, then write that down. Tell the universe that you want meaningful, inspirational and beautiful relationships by claiming that you already have them. In addition, you can visualize yourself ridding your life of toxic people who drag you down or make you feel badly about yourself.

Career and Creativity

Most working Americans spend more time at their jobs than they do anywhere else, so feeling satisfied with your profession can have a major impact on how you feel about your life and self-worth. Many people consider their vocation just a means to an end and settle for less than what they would love. But in reality, we are all born to be creative beings and bring forth our gifts. There is a school of thought dating all the way back to the Biblical times that says, if you don't express what is inside you it will eventually consume you. I believe this is true and that your ability to be creative directly affects your happiness and health.

Now, I am certainly not telling you to go and quit your day job tomorrow, but too many of us live our entire lives believing we are victims of our circumstances. To avoid doing this, when you create your dream life, ask yourself: What would I do if education, experience, money, fear or anything else were not a factor? Your answer to that question is your true calling and purpose in life. It is what your soul was meant to express. If you ignore this, you are stifling an extremely powerful inner energy, and it will eventually cause you unhappiness and dis-ease.

Finances

While doing what you love to do is important for self-fulfi   t, no one can ignore the fact that everyone needs money to survive. The good news is they are often connected. If you are doing something you love to do and you do it well, you are much more likely to succeed financially.

Money is just another form of energy, and the degree to which it flows into your life is representative of the good we bring into our lives and the lives of others. If the flow is not what you want it to be, then you need to visualize what you would love and bring those gifts that only you can bring into the world. If you do this, that energy will flow back into your life in the form of money.

When you write down your dream, do not forget to include this all-important detail. Write down where you would realistically like to be with your finances. Be specific when you are defining this. Write down exact salaries, write that your debts have zero balances, and exact material resources that you and your family and friends enjoy.

GETTING STARTED

Go buy a journal. It does not have to be fancy. And start writing down your dreams, in great detail. Focus on this dream, act as if it's already happened and I promise you will see vast improvements to your life.

When I first wanted to close my mainstream GYN practice and start this alternative practice, I read my dream over and over. I tweaked it and used it to manifest my life. It worked for me, and there's no reason why it won't work for you. I now use these tools with similar clients worldwide wanting to reinvent themselves and create lives they love living in my Midlife Diva coaching courses. (See resource section for further information).

BIKINI CODE BOTTOM LINE

It was when I was putting myself through this phase of the program that I decided to coin the term transformative health. And that's because I realized that this type of medicine was going to change my life and health—physically and mentally—forever. I would never go back because I was a different person. I had transformed into a new person, with a new understanding of my body, my health and my life. Other patients have had similar feelings. They tell me all the time that they feel like a completely different person, and that's what I mean when I say this medicine is truly transformative.

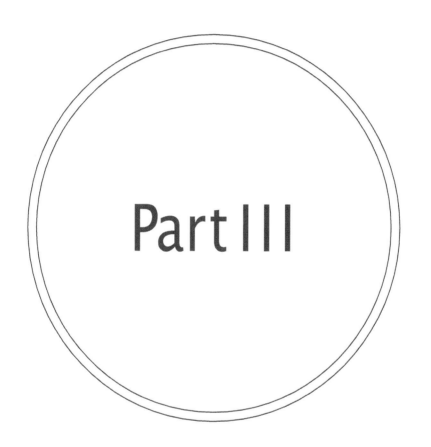

Part III

CHAPTER 12
Phase I Diet and Recipe Guide

T O HELP YOU CRACK THE BIKINI CODE ONCE AND FOR ALL, I have created an easy-to-follow diet plan and recipe guide. The following program details exactly what you should eat for breakfast, lunch, dinner and snacks for two weeks. Repeat this plan three times, and you will have made it through the six-week Phase I quick weight-loss program. Remember, you must take the recommended Phase I supplements with this program, and receive clearance from your personal physician before participating, otherwise you risk complications.

All the foods in this guide are guaranteed to help you nutrify and detoxify your body. However, this isn't your mother's diet food. Each one of these recipes has been handcrafted with your taste buds in mind. So, whether you are cooking for yourself—or a household of four—these recipes are guaranteed to please.

DAY 1

Breakfast:

Bikini Code Protein Shake (1 serving)

Cals: 123   carbs: 6   sugar: 0   fat: 14   protein: 2

1 3/4 ounce scoop Max Fit Protein Shake™
1 cup raw baby spinach, washed
4 strawberries
1 celery stalk
1 tablespoon MCT Oil Max™
1 5/8 ounce scoop Green Med™

Combine all of the ingredients together in a blender along with 1 cup ice and 1 cup water, and blend to your desired consistency.

Snack:

Simple Greek Salad (2 servings)

Cals: 52   carbs: 12   sugar: 3   fat: 0   protein: 2

1 whole cucumber, sliced or coarsely chopped
1 cup tomatoes, large dice
1 cup red onions, thinly sliced
2 tablespoons HCG Perfect Portions® Italian dressing*
1 tablespoon apple cider vinegar*

Combine the cucumbers, tomatoes, and onions in a mixing bowl. Lightly toss with the dressing and vinegar before eating.

The extra salad serving and the dressing may be refrigerated, covered, for 2 days.

Lunch:

Leafy Green Salad with Boiled Eggs (2 servings)

Cals: 136   carbs: 9   sugar: 2   fat: 5   protein: 10

2 boiled eggs, sliced
4 cups leafy greens of your choice
1/2 cup cucumber, coarsely chopped or sliced
1/2 cup tomato, large dice
1 tablespoon dressing of your choice

Fill a medium saucepan about halfway with water. Place the eggs in the water, cover, and bring to a boil over high heat. Once the water begins to boil, turn off the heat, but leave the pan on the burner. Let the eggs cool in the hot water until they have reached room temperature, then slice and serve over a bed of greens and vegetables that have been tossed with the salad dressing.

The extra salad serving may be kept covered, without dressing, in the refrigerator for 1 day.

Snack:

1 cup of strawberries (8 count) (1 serving)
Green Med™

Cals: 45   carbs: 11   sugar: 7   fat: 0   protein: 1

Dinner:

Beef (or Chicken) Bikini Wraps (4 servings)

BEEF: Cals: 321 carbs: 7 sugar: 4 fat: 15 protein: 28
CHICKEN: Cals: 263 carbs: 7 sugar: 4 fat: 5 protein: 34

1 tablespoon MCT Oil Max™*
4 (3.5 ounce-portions) chicken or beef, sliced or cubed
10 to 12 radishes, finely chopped
12 scallions, thinly sliced
2 cloves garlic, minced or thinly sliced
1/2 cup minced onion
1 cup chicken broth
4 tablespoons, Bragg's® Liquid Amino Acids*
8 large leaves lettuce, or cabbage

Heat the MCT oil in a large frying pan over medium heat and sauté the meat and vegetables for 5 minutes. Add the chicken broth and the Bragg's® Liquid Amino Acids and continue to cook until the vegetables and meat are done, about 8 to 10 minutes. Carefully spoon the meat mixture onto the center of each cabbage or lettuce leaf, wrap tightly and serve hot. The cooked meat portions of the Bikini Wraps may be frozen and reheated, but the lettuce needs to be fresh.

DAY 2

Breakfast:

I orange (1 serving)

Cals: 53 carbs: 13 sugar: 11 fat: 0 protein: 1

Snack:

10 to 12 gluten-free pretzels (1 serving)

Cals: 140 carbs: 0 sugar: 0 fat: 0 protein: 0

Lunch:

Skinny Sea Bass and Sautéed Spinach (4 servings)

Cals: 184 carbs: 5 sugar: 0 fat: 6 protein: 30

I teaspoon MCT Oil Max™*
4 (3.5-ounce) sea bass, tilapia, or cod fillets
2 tablespoons ginger, sliced
I clove garlic, minced or thinly sliced
I white onion, chopped
Fresh cilantro, to taste
4 cups fresh spinach leaves
I cup chicken stock

In a large frying pan, heat the MCT oil over medium-high heat and sear the sea bass on both sides until brown, about 3 minutes per side. Remove the fish from the pan, and add the ginger, garlic, onion, and cilantro to the remaining oil. Sauté, stirring, for 1 to 2 minutes, then add the spinach. Return the fish to the pan, add the chicken stock, and cover. Cook for 15 to 20 minutes. Serve the fish on a bed of vegetables.

Snack:

Fruit Salad (4 servings)

Cals: 46   carbs: 10   sugar: 7   fat: 0   protein: 1

2 cucumbers, diced
1 cup strawberries, diced
1 orange, peeled and diced
1 scoop Green Med™, or 1 packet Stevia
Juice of 1/2 lemon

Mix all the ingredients together, cover, and refrigerate before serving.
Extra portions may be refrigerated, covered, for up to 4 days.

Dinner:

Grilled Chicken Tenders with Asparagus Pesto (4 servings)

Cals: 105   carbs: 3   sugar: 1   fat: 10   protein: 23

4 (3.5-ounce) chicken brests, sliced in 1-inch strips
1 batch of Asparagus Pesto

Asparagus Pesto
8 to 10 asparagus tips
1 tablespoon red onion, minced
1 garlic clove, crushed or minced
2 teaspoons lemon juice
Pinch of sea salt
Cracked pepper to taste
2 tablespoons MCT Oil Max™

Preheat your oven to 350 degrees F.

To make the Asparagus Pesto, puree all ingredients in a blender or food processor.

If you wish to marinate the chicken in the pesto before cooking, brush the pesto over the chicken strips, cover and refrigerate for several hours. If you do not marinate the chicken, then spoon the pesto over the chicken just before cooking. Place the chicken strips on a baking sheet and bake for 20 minutes, turning after 10 minutes.

DAY 3

Breakfast:

1/2 grapefruit (1 serving)

Cals: 40 carbs: 10 sugar: 9 fat: 0 protein: 1

Snack:

Celery Sticks with Salsa (4 servings)

Skinny Salsa
5 Roma tomatoes, finely diced
1 small onion, finely diced
1/2 jalapeno, seeded and minced (add more if you like spicier salsa)
1 to 2 cloves garlic, minced
1/2 tablespoon fresh cilantro leaves
1/4 teaspoon cayenne pepper
Sea salt to taste
Juice of 1/2 lime
1 teaspoon lemon juice
2 stalks celery, cut into 1/4-inch sticks

Mix all salsa ingredients, except the celery sticks, together in a small bowl and refrigerate.

Serve chilled with the celery sticks.

Keep leftover salsa refrigerated for up to 3 days.

Lunch:

Better Body Meatballs with Marinara Sauce (4 servings)

Cals: 155   carbs: 7   sugar: 3   fat: 5   protein: 22

14 ounces ground lean beef, veal or chicken breast
1/2 teaspoon Onion & Herb Mrs. Dash®
4 gluten-free pretzels, crushed
1/2 clove garlic, minced
1 tablespoon onion, minced
1/2 cup marinara sauce, your choice brand
2 cups shredded cabbage

Preheat the oven to 350 degrees F.

In a large bowl, mix together the ground meat, Onion & Herb Mrs. Dash®, pretzels, garlic and onion. Form the mixture into 2-inch balls, place them in a baking dish, and cover with the marinara sauce. Bake for 25 to 30 minutes.

While the meatballs are cooking, place the cabbage in a medium saucepan, cover with water, and steam for 8 to 10 minutes, until the cabbage has softened. Serve the meatballs over the steamed cabbage.

Snack:

Fruit Salad (1 serving) (see p. 108 for recipe)

Dinner:

Carefree Cream of Chicken Soup (4 servings)

Cals: 56   carbs: 3   sugar: 1   fat: 3   protein: 22

4 (3.5-ounce) cooked chicken breasts, cut into ½-inch cubes
4 celery stalks, chopped, and leaves
1/2 cup onion, minced
1 garlic clove
1 teaspoon Mrs. Dash® Garlic & Herb
Sea salt to taste

Combine all the ingredients with 4 cups water in a food processor and blend until smooth. Pour the mixture into a large saucepan and simmer over medium heat for 20 minutes.

When you are ready to serve, add a celery leaf to garnish.

Refrigerate leftover soup in a container with a tight cover for up to 2 days. May freeze for 2 weeks.

DAY 4

Breakfast:

Sassy Cinnamon Apple Sauce (1 serving)

Cals: 103   carbs: 33   sugar: 6   fat: 0   protein: 1

1 large Granny Smith apple, cored and chopped
1/2 teaspoon ground cinnamon
Pinch of Stevia
1 celery stalk

Put all the ingredients along with 2 tablespoons water into a blender or food processor and puree.

May be refrigerated before serving, or enjoy at room temperature.

Snack:

Tiny Waist Thai Slaw (2 servings)

Cals: 18   carbs: 3   sugar: 1   fat: 0   protein: 1

½ cup diced radishes
1/8 cup minced onion
1/4 cup shredded green cabbage
1/4 cup shredded purple cabbage
1/8 teaspoon crushed red pepper flakes
1/8 teaspoon freshly grated ginger
Pinch of Stevia
1 tablespoon lemon juice
2 tablespoons apple cider vinegar

In a large mixing bowl, toss all the ingredients together. Refrigerate the slaw before serving.

The extra servings may be refrigerated in a covered container for up to 3 days.

Lunch:

Beach-Ready Crab Bisque (4 servings)

Cals: 57   carbs: 2   sugar: 2   fat: 2   protein: 6

4 ounces fresh or canned crabmeat
1 clove garlic
3 (6-inch) celery stalks
1/2 large onion, cut into chunks
2 medium tomatoes
3 tablespoons lemon juice
1 teaspoon Old Bay® seasoning
Cayenne pepper to taste

Put all the ingredients, except the crabmeat, in a food processor and blend until smooth. In a large saucepan over medium-high heat, stir the vegetable mixture together with the crabmeat and cook until it starts to boil, then turn the heat to low, and simmer for 10 minutes.

Leftover bisque servings can be frozen in airtight containers.

Snack:

10 to 12 gluten-free pretzels (1 serving)

Dinner:

Mediterranean Chicken and Vegetables (4 servings)

Cals: 138   carbs: 8   sugar: 3   fat: 4   protein: 19

1 tablespoon MCT Oil Max™
4 (3.5-ounce) chicken tenderloins, cubed
1 cup onion, chopped
16 grape tomatoes, halved
4 cups fresh spinach leaves

Heat the oil in a large frying pan over medium-high heat, and sauté the chicken, onion and tomatoes, stirring, for 10 minutes, or until the chicken is thoroughly cooked. Add 1 cup water and the spinach to the pan, and turn the heat to medium-low, cover and simmer for 3 to 5 minutes. Serve hot.

Extra servings can be refrigerated, covered, for up to 3 days.

DAY 5

Breakfast:

Sexy Sweet Ginger Smoothie (1 serving)

Cals: 46   carbs: 5   sugar: 2   fat: 0   protein: 0

4 strawberries
1/2 orange, peeled
1 scoop of Green Med™
¼ teaspoon ground ginger

Put all of the ingredients together in a blender with 1 cup ice and 6 to 8 ounces water and mix until you reach your desired consistency.

Snack:

Cucumbers

Lunch:

Garlic Shrimp with Sautéed Vegetables (4 servings)

Cals: 88   carbs: 5   sugar: 0   fat: 4   protein: 10

1 tablespoon MCT Oil Max™
12 medium or 6 jumbo shrimp
1 white onion, diced
10 cups spinach leaves
3 tablespoons Bragg's® Amino Acids*
1 teaspoon freshly ground ginger
1/2 teaspoon Garlic & Herb Mrs. Dash®

Heat the oil in a large frying pan over medium-high heat and sauté the shrimp for 7 to 8 minutes, turning, until thoroughly cooked. Add the remaining ingredients and 1 cup water, turn the heat to low, cover and simmer for 15 minutes.

Snack:

Bikini-Worthy Baked Apple Crumbles (2 servings)

Cals: 82   carbs: 18   sugar: 9   fat: 3   protein: 1

I teaspoon MCT or coconut oil*
4 gluten-free Melba rounds, crushed
I Granny Smith apple, chopped into 1-inch chunks
I packet Stevia
1/2 teaspoon pumpkin spice

Preheat your oven to 350 degrees F. Lightly coat a small oven-safe dish with MCT or coconut oil. Place the crushed Melba rounds to cover the bottom of the dish, then layer the apple chunks on top. Sprinkle the Stevia and pumpkin spice on the apples, and bake for 10 to 15 minutes.

Refrigerate, covered, for 2 days, or freeze in an airtight container for up to two weeks.

Dinner:

Code Cracking Chili (4 servings)

Cals: 160   carbs: 4   sugar: 2   fat: 7   protein: 20

14 ounces lean ground beef, veal or chicken
2 tablespoons onion, chopped
2 cloves garlic, minced
1/2 teaspoon chili powder
1/4 teaspoon garlic powder
I cup Roma tomatoes, diced
1/4 jalapeno pepper, minced (or more if you want more heat)

In a large frying pan over medium-high heat, brown the meat with the onions, garlic and dry spices. Add the tomatoes, jalapeno and ½ cup of water, then cover the pan, lower the heat to medium-low and simmer for 20 to 25 minutes.

Extra servings may be frozen in an airtight container.

DAY 6

Breakfast:

Figure-Flattering Frittata (1 serving)

Cals: 135 carbs: 7 sugar: 1 fat: 9 protein: 17

2 egg whites
1 tablespoon salsa (see p. xx for recipe)
1 cup spinach leaves, chopped
4 cherry tomatoes, cut in half
2 teaspoons MCT Oil Max™

Preheat your oven to 400 degrees F.

In a small bowl, stir together all the ingredients except the oil.

Coat an oven-safe omelet pan with MCT oil, pour in the egg mixture and bake, uncovered, for 12 to 15 minutes, or until it is golden brown on top.

Snack:

1 Granny Smith apple (1 serving)

Cals: 80 carbs: 22 sugar: 17 fat: 0 protein: 0

Lunch:

Tasty Tomato Soup (4 servings)

Cals: 167   carbs: 23   sugar: 17   fat: 1   protein: 6

4 cups Roma tomatoes, chopped
6 ounces tomato paste
8 fresh basil leaves, torn
2 cloves garlic
1/2 teaspoon Mrs. Dash® Italian Seasoning
2 cups chicken broth
Salt and pepper to taste

Combine all the ingredients along with 2 cups water in a food processor and puree. Pour the mixture into a saucepan over medium heat and simmer for 20 minutes.

Refrigerated servings may be kept, covered, for up to 2 days, but this soup does not freeze well.

Snack:

1 hard-boiled egg (1 serving)

Cals: 70   carbs: 1   sugar: 0   fat: 5   protein: 6

Dinner:

Apple and Herb Stuffed Chicken (4 servings)

Cals: 85   carbs: 4   sugar: 3   fat: 6   protein: 22

1/2 Granny Smith apple
1/2 medium red onion, chopped
1 tablespoon MCT Oil Max™
1/2 teaspoon Mrs. Dash® Garlic & Herb seasoning
Sea salt to taste
4 (3.5-ounce) chicken breasts

Pre-heat your oven to 350 degrees F.

In a small mixing bowl, stir together all ingredients, except the chicken.

Cut the chicken breasts in half and stuff the mixture into each of the 4 chicken breasts. Secure the stuffed breasts with a toothpick to close during baking.

Place the chicken on a small baking dish and bake, uncovered, for 30 to 35 minutes.

Extra servings may be refrigerated, covered, for up to 2 days.

DAY 7

Breakfast:

I cup strawberries (about 8) (1 serving)

Snack:

Simple Greek Salad (2 servings)

I whole cucumber, chopped
I cup tomatoes, coarsely chopped
I cup red onion, diced
2 tablespoons fat-free Italian dressing
I tablespoon apple cider vinegar

Toss all the vegetables in a mixing bowl with the dressing and vinegar.

The extra serving may be refrigerated overnight in a covered container.

Lunch:

Grilled Chicken Tenders with Asparagus Pesto (4 servings)

Cals: 105 carbs: 3 sugar: 1   fat: 10 protein: 23

I batch Asparagus Pesto (See p. 108 for recipe)
4 (3.5-ounce) chicken breasts, thickly sliced

Preheat your oven to 350 degrees F.

To make the Asparagus Pesto, puree all ingredients in a blender or food processor. You may marinate the chicken in the pesto sauce for a few hours, or you can simply brush it over the chicken just before cooking.

Place the chicken pieces on a baking sheet and bake for 20 minutes.

Extra servings of the chicken may be kept, covered and refrigerated, for up to 2 days.

Snack:

Tiny Waist Thai Slaw (1 serving) (See p. 112 for recipe)

Dinner:

Chicken Gumbo (4 servings)

Cals: 114 carbs: 10 sugar: 5 fat: 7 protein: 25

1 tablespoon MCT Oil Max™
10 to 12 asparagus cut into ¼-inch pieces
1 onion, chopped
4 cloves garlic, minced
4 (3.5-ounce) chicken breasts
1 tablespoon Creole seasoning
2 large tomatoes, diced
1 tablespoon tomato paste
2 cups organic low sodium chicken broth
Cayenne pepper and salt to taste

In a large frying pan over medium heat, sauté the asparagus, onion, and garlic in the oil for 3 to 5 minutes, until soft. Add the chicken and continue to cook for 8 to 10 minutes, turning, until brown on both sides. Sprinkle with the Creole seasoning, then stir in the tomatoes, tomato paste and chicken broth. Cover, turn the heat to medium-low, and simmer for 15 minutes more.

Extra servings may be frozen until you are ready to use.

DAY 8

Breakfast:

Bikini Body Protein Shake (1 serving) (See p. 104 for recipe)

Snack:

Celery Sticks with Salsa (1 serving) (see p. 109 for recipe)

Lunch:

Leafy Green Salad with Boiled Eggs (1 serving) (see p. 105 for recipe)

Snack:

1 cup strawberries (about 8) (1 serving)
1 orange

Dinner:

Grilled Chicken with Sweet Onions (4 servings)

Cals: 126   carbs: 6   sugar: 5   fat: 4   protein: 19

1 tablespoon MCT Oil Max™
4 (3.5-ounce) chicken tenderloins
2 sweet Vidalia onions, sliced in rings
1 tablespoon Mrs. Dash® Garlic and Herb
1/2 packet of Stevia, or to taste

Heat the MCT oil in a large frying pan over medium-high heat and sauté the chicken for 8 to 10 minutes, turning, until brown on both sides. Add the onions, spices, and 2 tablespoons water, turn the heat to low, and simmer, covered, for 15 to 20 minutes, or until tender.

Extra servings of the chicken may be refrigerated in a covered container for 2 days.

DAY 9

Breakfast:

I cup strawberries (about 8) (1 serving)

Snack:

Simple Greek Salad (1 serving) (see p. 104 for recipe)

Lunch:

Better Body Meatballs with Marinara Sauce (1 serving)
(see p. 110 for recipe)

Snack:

Fruit Salad (1 serving) (see p. 108 for recipe)

Dinner:

Grilled Chicken Tenders with Asparagus Pesto (1 serving)
(see p. 108 for recipe)

DAY 10

Breakfast:

Fruit Salad (1 serving) (see p. 108 for recipe)

Snack:

Cucumbers (1 serving)

Lunch:

Tilapia Tuna-Style Salad (4 servings)

Cals: 100   carbs: 0   sugar: 0   fat: 2   protein: 20

I batch Relish, recipe below
5 cups shredded cabbage
4 (3.5-ounce) tilapia fillets

Relish
1 cucumber, minced
¼ cup apple cider vinegar
1 teaspoon ground mustard
1 teaspoon dill
¼ teaspoon allspice
½ packet Stevia
½ teaspoon sea salt

Mix all the relish ingredients in a bowl and transfer the mixture to a covered jar or container, and refrigerate for 2 to 3 hours. If you prefer, you can puree the mixture to achieve a smooth appearance.

Extra servings may be kept, covered, in the refrigerator for up to 2 days.

Snack:

8 Melba Rounds with **Skinny Salsa** (1 serving) (see p. 109 for recipe)

Dinner:

Grilled Beef Fajitas (4 servings)

Cals: 157   carbs: 2   sugar: 27   fat: 7   protein: 28

1 tablespoon MCT Oil Max™
1/2 white onion, chopped
1 banana pepper, sliced
4 (3.5-ounce) tenderloin, flank or round beef cuts, sliced into 3-inch strips
½ teaspoon Mrs. Dash® Fajita Seasoning Mix
4 lime wedges

Heat the oil in a large frying pan over medium heat, and sauté the onions and peppers. Add the beef and seasoning and continue stirring for 8 to 10 minutes, or until the beef is fully cooked.

Squeeze a little lime juice on the beef before you serve.

DAY 11

Breakfast:

1/2 grapefruit

Snack:

1 cup strawberries (about 8)

Lunch:

Beef Kabobs (4 servings)

Cals: 147   carbs: 11   sugar: 8   fat: 2   protein: 19

4 (3.5-ounce) flank steaks or tenderloins, cubed
2 cups pearl onions
4 cups cherry tomatoes
4 tablespoons Bragg's Liquid Amino Acids*
1 tablespoon Mrs. Dash Steak Seasoning

In large dish, marinate the meat with the Liquid Amino Acids and steak seasoning for at least 20 minutes, or cover and marinate overnight in the refrigerator. When you are ready to cook, divide the meat and vegetables into 4 portions, skewer each portion, and grill. If you don't have access to a grill, place the skewers in a shallow pan under the broiler, and cook 3 to 5 minutes on each side.

Snack:

Simple Greek Salad (2 servings) (see p. 104 for recipe)

Dinner:

Skinny Sea Bass and Sautéed Spinach (see p. 107 for recipe)

DAY 12

Breakfast:

1 to 1 Spinach Omelet

Cals: 202   carbs: 9   sugar: 4   fat: 18   protein: 12

1 whole egg
1 egg white
Salt and pepper to taste
1 tablespoon MCT oil*
1 cup fresh baby spinach leaves
2 tablespoons salsa (see p. xx for recipe)

In a small bowl, beat the egg, egg white, salt and pepper together with a fork.

Heat the oil in a frying pan over medium-low heat, and carefully pour the egg mixture into the pan. Let the egg cook for 2 to 3 minutes, then carefully place the spinach and salsa in middle of the omelet. Use a spatula to remove the omelet from the pan and fold over to serve.

Snack:

10 to 12 gluten-free pretzels

Lunch:

Strawberry Salad (2 servings)

Cals: 115   carbs: 1   sugar: 0   fat: 1   protein: 24

2 (3.5-ounce) chicken tenders
1 tablespoon no- or low-sodium poultry seasoning
4 cups raw spinach, washed
1/8 cup chopped cilantro
1 cup (about 8) strawberries, diced
4 tablespoons Strawberry Vinaigrette*

Preheat your oven to 350 degrees F.

Rinse and dry the chicken tenderloins and season on both sides. Place the chicken on a baking sheet and bake for 20 minutes, turning after 10 minutes to brown both sides.

In a medium mixing bowl, mix the spinach and cilantro together.

To serve, toss the greens with the Strawberry Vinaigrette dressing and serve the chicken on top of the salad.

For the extra serving, the spinach and cilantro mixture must be refrigerated separately from the strawberries, dressing and the chicken, and will keep, refrigerated, for up to 2 days. Assemble when ready to serve. Do not freeze.

Strawberry Vinaigrette (4 servings)
4 tablespoons Perfect Portions® Vinaigrette
4 strawberries

Mix all ingredients in a blender until smooth. Will keep in refrigerator, covered, for 1 week.

Snack:

1 boiled egg with salsa (1 serving) (see p. 109 for recipe)

Dinner:

Chicken Curry Soup (4 servings)

Cals: 127   carbs: 11   sugar: 4   fat: 7   protein: 25

I teaspoon MCT Oil Max™
1/2 Granny Smith apple, thinly sliced
1/2 fennel bulb, thinly sliced
1/2 onion, thinly sliced
I clove garlic
I tablespoon curry powder
4 (3.5-ounce) chicken breasts, cut into ½-inch cubes
4 cups chicken broth

Heat the oil in a large frying pan over medium heat. Sauté the apple, fennel, onion, and garlic for 3 to 5 minutes, until tender, and stir in the curry powder. Add the chicken and sauté for 6 to 8 minutes, turning until both sides are brown. Add the chicken broth, cover, lower the heat and simmer for 10 to 15 minutes, until the chicken is tender.

Extra servings may be kept, covered, in the refrigerator for up to 2 days, or frozen in an airtight container for 2 weeks.

DAY 13

Breakfast:

Bikini-Worthy Baked Apple Crumbles (1 serving)
(see p. 116 for recipe)

Snack:

Fruit Salad (1 serving) (see p. 108 for recipe)

Lunch:

Grilled BBQ Chicken Salad (2 servings)

Cals: 123   carbs: 2   sugar: 21   fat: 2   protein: 24

2 (3.5-ounce) chicken tenderloins
1/2 cup HCG Perfect Portions® BBQ Sauce*
4 to 6 cups leafy greens
1/4 cup red onion, sliced
1/4 cup Sweet Mustard Vinaigrette (see p. 131 for recipe)

Preheat your grill to 350 degrees F, or use the broiler of your oven to cook the chicken.

Coat the chicken with BBQ sauce and grill, turning, for 10 to 12 minutes until brown on all sides. Allow the chicken to cool enough to handle. Once cooled, cut the chicken into ½-inch slices.

Toss the greens with the onions and Sweet Mustard Vinaigrette dressing. Serve the chicken on top of the greens.

For the extra serving, keep the chicken, greens and onion separately in the refrigerator, covered, then assemble when you are ready to serve. Do not freeze.

Sweet Mustard Vinaigrette (4 servings)
4 tablespoons Perfect Portions® Vinaigrette
I teaspoon mustard seed powder

Mix all ingredients in with a whisk in a bowl until blended. Will keep in refrigerator, covered, for 2 weeks.

Snack:

Celery Sticks with Salsa (1 serving) (see p. 109 for recipe)

Dinner:

Garlic Shrimp with Sautéed Vegetables (1 serving)
(see p. 115 for recipe)

DAY 14

Breakfast:

Fruit Salad (1 serving) (see p. 108 for recipe)

Snack:

Sautéed Vegetables (4 servings)

Cals: 369   carbs: 61   sugar: 15   fat: 26   protein: 10

1 tablespoon MCT Oil Max™
2 cups asparagus, sliced into 1-inch pieces
2 cups onions, sliced
2 cups spinach leaves
2 cups shredded cabbage
2 cloves garlic, minced
Mrs. Dash® Garlic & Herb to taste

Heat the oil in a large frying pan over medium heat. Sauté all the vegetables for 10 minutes, or until tender.

Lunch:

Leafy Green Salad with Boiled Eggs (1 serving)
(see p. 105 for recipe)

Snack:

Bikini Code Protein Shake (1 serving) (see p. 104 for recipe)

Dinner:

Grilled Chicken Fajitas (4 servings)

Cals: 144   carbs: 2   sugar: 1   fat: 5   protein: 23

1 tablespoon MCT Oil Max™
½ white onion, chopped
1 banana pepper, sliced
4 (3.5-ounce) chicken breasts, cubed
1/2 teaspoon Mrs Dash® Fajita Seasoning Mix
4 lime wedges

Heat the oil in a large frying pan over medium heat, and sauté the onions and peppers for 3 to 5 minutes. Add the chicken and fajita seasoning and continue cooking for 8 to 10 minutes, stirring, until the chicken is fully cooked. Squeeze a little lime juice on the chicken when ready to serve.

Extra servings may be frozen in airtight containers.

CHAPTER 13
Phase II Diet and Recipe Guide

FOR PHASE II, I ASKED CHEF BRYAN GRAVES TO SHARE some of his tastiest meals with you. During this phase you have much more lenience on which days you eat what, but here are dozens of recipes that will help you stay on track.

For convenience, I asked Bryan to create meals that consisted of up to four servings. You can share them with your family, keep them in the refrigerator for up to 3 days or freeze the extras for another day. When storing, be sure to seal the vegetables in a separate container from the meat.

Chicken Breast with Mustard Greens
and Fennel Orange Slaw (4 servings)

Cals: 375   carbs: 28   sugar: 15   fat: 14   protein: 44

1 tablespoon fresh thyme, chopped
1 tablespoon parsley, chopped
1 tablespoon lemon juice
1 tablespoon, plus 3 teaspoons olive oil
Salt and pepper
4 (6-ounce) boneless chicken breasts
3 bunches mustard greens, coarsely chopped
2 fennel bulbs, thinly sliced
Juice and zest of 1 orange
1 can mandarin oranges, drained
1 tablespoon cilantro, chopped
1 teaspoon ginger, pureed

In a large bowl, combine the thyme, parsley, lemon juice, 1 teaspoon olive oil, salt and pepper and marinate the chicken, covered, in the refrigerator for two hours.

Preheat your oven to 350 degrees F.

Heat 1 tablespoon olive oil in a medium sauté pan on medium-high heat and sauté the chicken for 3 to 5 minutes on each side, until golden brown.

Transfer the chicken to a roasting pan and bake, uncovered, for 5 to 8 minutes until done. Remove from the oven and cover to keep warm while you cook the mustard greens.

Heat 1 teaspoon olive oil in a stockpot over high heat, and stir in the mustard greens to coat them with the oil, and cook for 2 to 3 minutes. Add 2 cups water and reduce the heat to medium-low. Cover and cook for 15 to 20 minutes, stirring every 5 minutes. Season with salt and pepper to taste.

To make the fennel relish, combine the fennel in a mixing bowl with the orange juice and zest, the mandarin oranges, cilantro, ginger, 1 teaspoon olive oil, and salt and pepper to taste.

Arrange the mustard greens on a plate with a sliced chicken breast. Put a portion of the fennel relish on each chicken breast.

Extra servings can be refrigerated, in separate covered containers for the relish and chicken, and kept for up to 3 days.

Pork Tenderloin with Edamame Relish and Roasted Yellow Squash (4 Servings)

Cals: 415   carbs: 17   sugar: 5   fat: 16   protein: 48

1 tablespoon rosemary, chopped
Salt and pepper
3 teaspoons olive oil
1 (2-pound) pork tenderloin
2 pounds yellow squash, diced
1 tablespoon thyme, chopped
2 cups edamame beans, blanched
1 tablespoon lemon juice
1/4 cup chopped basil

Combine the rosemary, salt, pepper and 1 teaspoon olive oil, and marinate the pork in a bowl or pan, covered, for 4 hours or overnight, in the refrigerator.

Preheat your oven to 350 degrees F.

When you are ready to cook, pat the pork tenderloin dry with paper towels and season with salt and pepper. Heat a large sauté pan on medium-high and sear the pork on all sides until golden brown. This will take about 5 minutes. Transfer the pork to a roasting pan and roast for 10 to 15 minutes, or until the meat reaches an internal temperature of 160 degrees F for medium, or 145 degrees F for medium-rare. Remove from the oven and let the pork rest for 10 minutes at room temperature before slicing and serving.

Place the diced squash in a large mixing bowl. Stir in 1 teaspoon olive oil, thyme, salt, pepper and mix well. Transfer this mixture to a separate roasting pan and bake for 12 to 15 minutes.

In a small bowl, combine the edamame, lemon juice, basil, salt, pepper and 1 teaspoon olive oil and mix well.

Arrange the baked squash on a plate with the sliced pork. Spoon the edamame relish atop the pork and serve.

Extra servings can be covered and kept in the refrigerator for 3 to 4 days.

Grilled Pork Chops with Baby Carrots and Arugula

(4 servings)

Cals: 528   carbs: 18   sugar: 10   fat: 30   protein: 47

2 teaspoons olive oil
1 tablespoon fresh orange juice with 1 tablespoon zest, divided
1 tablespoon fresh thyme, chopped
1 teaspoon roasted garlic puree (see p. 164 for recipe)
Salt and pepper
1 tablespoon parsley, chopped
4 (6-ounce) boneless pork chops
1 1/2 pounds baby carrots, peeled
8 ounces arugula

In a large bowl, combine 1 teaspoon olive oil, orange zest, thyme, roasted garlic puree, salt, pepper, parsley and marinate the chops, covered, for 4 hours, or overnight in the refrigerator.

Heat your grill to 350 degrees F. Grill the pork chops for 5 to 6 minutes on each side, or until they reach an internal temperature of 160 degrees F. Allow the meat to rest 10 minutes before serving.

Blanch the carrots in boiling salted water for 4 minutes, then drain on a paper towel. Heat 1 teaspoon of oil in a medium sauté pan over medium-high heat and add the blanched carrots. Season with salt and pepper, and cook for 2 minutes, or until tender.

In a medium mixing bowl, toss together the arugula, orange juice, 1 teaspoon olive oil, salt and pepper.

Plate the carrots, place the pork chop on top of them and add the arugula on top of the chops.

Extra servings can be covered and kept in the refrigerator for 3 to 4 days.

Herb-Crusted Rack of Lamb with Collards and Toasted Cashews (4 servings)

Cals: 573   carbs: 12   sugar: 4   fat: 48   protein: 36

1 tablespoon rosemary, chopped
1 tablespoon parsley, chopped
1 tablespoon fresh thyme, chopped
2 racks lamb (about 3 pounds)
2 bunches collard greens, cleaned and chopped
1 tablespoon plus 1 teaspoon olive oil
2 cups chicken stock
1 1/2 cups toasted cashews

Preheat your oven to 350 degrees F.

Mix the rosemary, parsley and thyme together in a bowl. Season all sides of the lamb with this herb mixture.

Heat 1 tablespoon olive oil in a medium sauté pan over medium-high heat and sear the lamb on both sides until golden brown. You may need to add extra oil.

Place the lamb in a roasting pan and bake for 12 to 15 minutes. Use a meat thermometer to check the internal temperature after 10 minutes: 135 degrees F, rare; 145 degrees F, medium rare; 155 degrees F, medium; 165 degrees F, well done.

Allow the lamb to rest for 10 minutes at room temperature before slicing. The meat will continue to cook for 5 to 10 degrees more after it is removed from the oven.

Slice the lamb between the bones.

Heat a medium stockpot over medium-high heat and add 1 teaspoon olive oil and the collards, stirring to coat the greens with the olive oil. Cook for 2 minutes and season with salt and pepper. Cook for an additional 2 minutes, then add the chicken stock, reduce the heat to medium-low and cover. Cook for another 20 minutes, stirring every 8 minutes or so.

In a small food processor, pulse the cashews about 3 times. Transfer to a bowl.

Plate the collards, arrange the lamb slices around the plate, and garnish with the cashew pieces.

Extra servings can be covered and kept in the refrigerator for 3 to 4 days.

Grilled Lamb Chops with Brussels Sprouts and Tomato-Mint Relish (4 servings)

Cals: 341 carbs: 23 sugar: 10 fat: 18 protein: 15

8 lamb loin chops (3 ½- ounces each)
Salt and pepper
1 1/2 pounds Brussels sprouts, trimmed and halved
1 tablespoon rosemary, chopped
1 tablespoon plus 1 teaspoon olive oil
1 teaspoon lemon juice
4 Roma tomatoes, diced
4 cups mint, chopped

Heat your grill to 350 degrees F.

Season the lamb chops generously with salt and pepper and grill on each side for 3 minutes for medium-rare.

Stir the Brussels sprout halves in a mixing bowl with rosemary, salt, pepper and 1 teaspoon olive oil. Transfer to a shallow pan and roast for 20 to 25 minutes until tender. Toss lemon juice before serving.

Put the tomatoes into a food processor and pulse 4 times. Add the mint and 1 teaspoon olive oil and pulse 4 more times.

Place the Brussels sprouts and the lamb on a serving plate and spoon the tomato-mint relish over the lamb.

Extra servings can be covered and kept in the refrigerator for 3 to 4 days.

Beef Flank Steak with Kale and Pineapple Salsa

(4 servings)

Cals: 342   carbs: 13   sugar: 10   fat: 15   protein: 37

1 (24-ounce) beef flank steak
Juice and zest of 2 limes, divided
2 tablespoons cilantro, chopped
1 teaspoon sesame oil
1 tablespoon ginger, pureed
1 teaspoon olive oil
2 bunches kale, chopped
2 cups chicken stock
1 pineapple, peeled, cored and diced
1/2 teaspoon cumin
1 teaspoon pureed garlic (see p. 164 for recipe)

Mix the juice and zest of 1 lime, 1 tablespoon cilantro, sesame oil and ginger, and marinate the steak for 2 hours, or overnight.

Heat your grill to 350 degrees F.

Season the steak generously with salt and pepper and grill each side for 3 to 4 minutes for medium-rare. Allow the steak to rest at room temperature for 5 to 10 minutes.

Heat 1 teaspoon olive oil in a medium stock pot over medium high heart and add the kale.

Cook for 2 minutes, stirring frequently. Season with salt and pepper and continue to cook for 2 more minutes. Add the chicken stock and reduce the heat to medium-low , cover and cook for another 10 minutes.

In a medium mixing bowl, combine the pineapple, cilantro, lime juice, cumin, garlic, salt, pepper, and mix well.

To serve, slice the steak against the grain. Place the kale in the center of the serving plate and layer the steak slices on top. Spoon the pineapple salsa over the steak.

Extra servings can be covered and kept in the refrigerator for 3 to 4 days.

Beef Tenderloin with Portobello Mushrooms, Roasted Tomatoes and White Asparagus (4 servings)

Cals: 345   carbs: 12   sugar: 5   fat: 20   protein: 4

Marinade
1 teaspoon basil, chopped
Pureed garlic (see p. 164 for recipe)
1 teaspoon lemon juice
1 teaspoon olive oil
Salt and pepper to taste

4 (5 to 6-ounce) beef tenderloins
1 pint cherry tomatoes
1 teaspoon olive oil
Salt and pepper to taste
1 teaspoon dried thyme

2 portabello mushrooms
1 tablespoon olive oil
2 cloves garlic, crushed

2 pounds white asparagus, trimmed
1 teaspoon olive oil
1 tablespoon walnuts, crushed

To make the marinade, add the basil and the garlic puree to a food processor and puree until smooth. Add the lemon juice and pulse twice. Drizzle 1 teaspoon olive oil with food processor running. Transfer the marinade to a bowl and season with salt and pepper.

Marinate the beef in the basil mixture for 4 hours or overnight. In the refrigerator, reserve 4 tablespoons of basil puree to serve with the steaks.

When you are ready to cook the beef, heat a grill to 350 degrees F.

Grill the steaks for 5 to 6 minutes on each side, depending on thickness of the meat. Check the internal temperature using a meat thermometer. Longer cooking times might be required. Temperatures for doneness are: 125 degrees F for rare; 140 degrees F for medium-rare; 145 degrees F for medium; 150 degrees F for medium-well; and 155 degrees F for well done.

Allow the steak to rest at room temperature for 10 minutes before serving.

When you are ready to cook the vegetables, preheat your oven to 250 degrees F.

Put the tomatoes in mixing bowl and stir together with 1 teaspoon olive oil, salt, pepper, and dried thyme. Transfer the tomatoes to a shallow pan and roast for 20 to 25 minutes.

To make the portobello mushrooms, remove the gills from the portabellos with a spoon and dice. Heat a large sauté pan over medium-high heat, add 1 tablespoon olive oil and the mushrooms and sauté for 4 minutes. Stir in the crushed garlic, season with salt and pepper and continue to cook for 3 minutes.

To make the asparagus, heat the olive oil in a medium sauté pan over medium heat and sauté the asparagus spears for 2 minutes. Season with salt and pepper and continue to cook 4 to 6 minutes, or until tender. Stir in the crushed walnuts.

Place the tomatoes and mushrooms in the center of the serving plate. Place the beef on top with the reserved basil puree. Arrange the asparagus spears around the sides.

Lobster, Shrimp, and Mussels
in Tomato Saffron Broth (4 servings)

Cals: 417   carbs: 29   sugar: 10   fat: 10   protein: 52

1 lobster tail
Salt and pepper
3 teaspoons olive oil
1 pound peeled medium shrimp
16 mussels
1 1/2 cups chicken broth
1/2 pint cherry tomatoes
1 tablespoon pureed garlic (see p. 164 for recipe)
1 (16-ounce) can crushed tomatoes
1 pinch saffron
1/4 cup chopped basil
1/4 cup chopped parsley

Preheat your oven to 350 degrees F.

Season the lobster with salt and pepper, then butterfly it. Use kitchen shears to cut through the top of the shell and through the meat, stopping before the bottom shell. Use your fingers to spread the shell to loosen it from the meat. Separate the meat with your thumbs and pry it from the bottom shell, leaving it attached near the back end. Pull the meat upward so that is partially above the shells' halves as it cooks.

Transfer to a roasting pan and roast for 15 to 20 minutes, then remove and allow to cool enough to handle. Remove the meat from the shell and dice. Set aside.

Heat 1 teaspoon olive oil in a medium sauté pan over high heat and add the shrimp. Season with salt and pepper, and cook for 90 seconds, stirring frequently. Move the shrimp to a large mixing bowl and set aside.

Using the same sauté pan, wipe clean, then heat 1 teaspoon olive oil over high heat and add the mussels, stirring to coat. Add ½ cup chicken stock and cover. Cook for 2 minutes, or until just the shells start to open. Remove from heat and add the mussels to the bowl of shrimp.

Heat 1 teaspoon of olive oil in a medium stockpot over medium-high heat and add the cherry tomatoes. Cook for 3 minutes, then add the garlic and stir. Add the crushed tomato, chicken stock and saffron, and reduce the heat to medium-low. Cover and cook for 10 minutes. Next add the shrimp, lobster, mussels, basil and parsley. Season with salt and pepper to taste and heat through before serving.

Flounder with Basil Walnut Pesto and Roasted Squash (4 servings)

Cals: 288   carbs: 8   sugar: 3   fat: 21   protein: 35

4 (6-ounce) portions flounder
Salt and pepper to tastes
1 1/2 pounds yellow squash, diced
1 teaspoon garlic, chopped
1 tablespoon parsley
1/4 cup plus 1 teaspoon olive oil
2 cloves garlic
1/2 cup walnuts, chopped
2 cups basil, chopped
1 teaspoon lemon juice

Preheat your oven to 350 degrees F.

Season the flounder generously on both sides with salt and pepper. Place in a shallow baking dish and bake for 8 to 10 minutes, or until fish is flaky and tender.

Place the diced squash in a large mixing bowl and add the chopped garlic, parsley, 1 teaspoon olive oil, salt, pepper and mix well. Transfer to a baking dish and roast the squash for 15 to 18 minutes, until tender.

To make the walnut pesto, puree the garlic in a food processor until smooth. Add the walnuts and pulse 3 times. Add the basil and pulse 1 time. Keeping the processor running, drizzle in ¼ cup olive oil until the mixture is smooth. Season with salt, pepper and lemon juice.

Arrange the squash on a plate, add the fish and top with the pesto sauce.

Sea Bass with Warm Black Bean Salad, Asparagus and Yellow Tomato Salsa Verde (4 servings)

Cals: 481   carbs: 11   sugar: 4   fat: 16   protein: 26

2 cans organic black beans, drained
I teaspoon ginger, diced
1 tablespoon red onion, diced finely
I tablespoon cilantro
I teaspoon cumin
I teaspoon lime juice
Salt and pepper

2 medium yellow tomatoes
I small white onion, diced
I clove garlic, peeled
I cup cilantro leaves
I teaspoon salt
I tablespoon olive oil

4 (6-ounce) sea bass fillets
Salt and pepper
I teaspoon olive oil

I pound asparagus, trimmed
I teaspoon olive oil
Salt and pepper to taste

Preheat your oven to 350 degrees F.

Put the black beans in a bowl and add the ginger, onion, cilantro, cumin, lime juice, salt, pepper and mix well. Set aside.

Heat a large sauté pan over high heat and add the tomatoes, onion and garlic, and cook for 10 minutes then remove the garlic and set aside. Continue to cook the tomato mixture for another 10 minutes, or until the tomatoes have charred.

Add the tomato mixture along with the garlic, cilantro, salt, a dash of pepper, and 2 tablespoons olive oil in a blender and blend until smooth.

Place the sea bass on a plate and pat dry on both sides with paper towels. Season both sides with salt and pepper.

Heat a medium sauté pan over medium-high heat. Add the olive oil and sauté the fish, 2 at a time, for 3 minutes on both sides, until golden brown. Transfer the fish to a baking sheet. Repeat with the last 2 fillets, then bake the fish for 6 to 8 minutes.

Heat 1 teaspoon olive oil in a large sauté pan on medium-high heat, add the asparagus and cook for 4 to 5 minutes. Season with salt and pepper and cover to keep warm until you are ready to serve.

Transfer the black beans to a saucepot and heat over medium heat until warm.

Spoon the beans onto a plate, add the fish and top with the tomato salsa verde. Garnish with the asparagus.

Grilled Mahi with Shiitake, White Bean Relish, and Sautéed Spinach (4 servings)

Cals: 371   carbs: 36   sugar: 5   fat: 9   protein: 40

4 (6-ounce) Mahi fillets
Salt and pepper
1 tablespoon olive oil
1 pound shiitake mushrooms, stemmed and sliced
1 teaspoon olive oil,
1 teaspoon pureed garlic (see p. 164 for recipe)
1 (12-ounce) can organic cannellini beans, strained and rinsed
1 tablespoon parsley, chopped
2 tablespoons lemon juice

¾ pound baby spinach leaves
1 teaspoon olive oil

Heat a grill to 350 degrees F.

Season the fillets on both sides with salt and pepper and grill for 4 to 5 minutes on each side.

Heat 1 tablespoon olive oil in a large sauté pan over medium-high heat, Add the sliced mushrooms and cook for 3 minutes. Add the garlic puree, stir, and cook for 3 minutes.

Stir the cannellini beans in a large bowl with the parsley, lemon juice, salt, pepper, and 1 teaspoon olive oil. Add the beans to the pan of mushrooms and cook over medium heat until heated through.

In a separate large sauté pan heat 1 teaspoon of olive oil over high heat and add the spinach, stirring until it has wilted.

Place the spinach on a plate with the Mahi on top. Add a portion of the mushroom and bean relish on top of the fish.

Seared Mahi with Roasted Zucchini and Sesame Swiss Chard Salad (4 servings)

Cals: 173   carbs: 0   sugar: 0   fat: 8   protein: 32

4 (6-ounce) Mahi fillets
Salt and pepper
I teaspoon olive oil

I 1/2 pounds zucchini, medium dice
I teaspoon olive oil
1 tablespoon fresh thyme, finely chopped
Salt and pepper

I bunch rainbow Swiss chard, cut into ¼-inch vertical strips
I teaspoon black sesame seeds
I teaspoon sesame oil
½ teaspoon pureed ginger
I pint cherry tomatoes, thinly sliced
Juice of I/2 orange

Preheat your oven to 350 degrees F.

Dry the Mahi on both sides with a paper towel and season with salt and pepper.

Heat a skillet with 1 teaspoon olive oil and sear the fish on both sides for 3 minutes, until golden brown. Transfer the fish to a baking sheet and bake for 8 to 10 minutes.

Put the diced zucchini in mixing bowl and stir together with the olive oil, thyme, salt and pepper. Transfer to a roasting pan and cook for 14 to 18 minutes, or until tender.

Toss the Swiss chard in a bowl with the sesame seeds, sesame oil, ginger, tomatoes and orange juice.

Serve the fish atop a bed of zucchini with the Swiss chard on the side.

Shrimp with Basil, Lemon, and Black Beans (4 servings)

Cals: 427   carbs: 31   sugar: 1   fat: 6   protein: 42   sodium: 718

1 tablespoon ginger pureed
2 tablespoons olive oil, divided
2 pounds medium shrimp, peeled and deveined
Salt and pepper
2 (12-ounce) cans black beans, drained and rinsed
1/4 cup chopped basil
1 tablespoon parsley, chopped
3 tablespoons fresh lemon juice

To make the ginger puree, place a 4-inch piece of fresh, peeled ginger into a food processor and puree.

Heat 1 tablespoon olive oil in a large sauté pan over medium-high heat and sauté the shrimp, ginger, salt and pepper, stirring frequently, for 3 to 4 minutes, until the shrimp are pink.

Strain and rinse the black beans in a colander. Heat in a saucepan until warm.

In a large bowl, combine the shrimp, black beans, basil, parsley, lemon juice, 1 tablespoon olive oil, salt and pepper. Mix well and serve.

Grilled Chicken Breast with Butternut Squash, Asparagus and Pear Relish (4 servings)

Cals: 432   carbs: 30   sugar: 21   fat: 14   protein: 37

4 (6-ounce) boneless chicken breasts, skin removed
1 tablespoon lime juice
1 tablespoon parsley
1 tablespoon rosemary, chopped
1 tablespoon olive oil
Salt and pepper

1 pound asparagus, trimmed

2 medium butternut squash, peeled and diced
1 teaspoon olive oil
Salt and pepper

3 pears, peeled, cored and diced
1 teaspoon olive oil
1/4 cup golden raisins
1 tablespoon chopped fresh sage
1 tablespoon chopped parsley
Salt and pepper

Combine the chicken in a bowl with the lime juice, parsley, rosemary, olive oil, salt and pepper. Cover and marinate for 4 hours, or up to 2 days in the refrigerator before cooking.

Preheat your oven to 350 degrees F and heat-up a grill to 350 degrees F.

Season the asparagus with salt and pepper and grill for 3 to 4 minutes, turning to cook evenly.

Grill the marinated chicken on both sides for 4 to 5 minutes, until done.

Place the squash in bowl with 1 teaspoon olive oil, salt and pepper, and mix thoroughly.

Transfer to a roasting pan and cook for 20 to 25 minutes, until tender.

Heat the diced pears with 1 teaspoon olive oil in a medium saucepan over medium heat.

Sauté the pears for 4 minutes, then add the raisins, sage, parsley, salt and pepper, and cook for 3 more minutes, stirring frequently. Remove from the heat and allow to cool to room temperature.

Slice the chicken breasts and arrange on a plate with the squash and asparagus. Top with the pear relish.

Pan-Sautéed Snapper with Green Beans and Ginger Papaya (4 servings)

Cals: 280   carbs: 14   sugar: 10   fat: 6   protein: 41

4 (6-ounce) snapper fillets
Salt and pepper

I pound green beans
I tablespoon kosher salt
I teaspoon olive oil

I 1/2 cups papaya pulp
I tablespoon ginger puree
I tablespoon chopped cilantro, plus more for garnish
I teaspoon oil

Preheat your oven to 350 degrees F.

Place the fish on a plate and pat both sides dry with paper towels. Season with salt and pepper. Heat 1 teaspoon olive oil in a large saucepan over medium-high heat and sear the fillets, two at a time, for 3 minutes on each side, until golden brown. Remove the fish to a baking sheet and repeat with the remaining two fillets. Bake the fish for 6 to 8 minutes, or until the meat is flaky.

Fill a large saucepan halfway with water and bring to a boil over high heat. Add the green beans and the kosher salt, and blanch the beans for 5 minutes. Drain and let sit for 1 minute to dry, then toss in a bowl with salt, pepper and 1 teaspoon olive oil.

To get the papaya pulp, cut the papaya open and deseed. Scoop out the pulp and roughly chop.

To puree the ginger, place a 4-inch piece of fresh, peeled ginger into a food processor and pulse to a desired consistency.

Add the papaya pulp, ginger puree, cilantro, and 1 teaspoon oil into a blender and blend until smooth.

Arrange the green beans on a plate and top with the snapper. Top with the papaya puree and garnish with cilantro.

Baked Grouper with Peach-Mint Relish
and Asparagus (4 servings)

Cals: 324   carbs: 19   sugar: 10   fat: 7   protein: 40

4 (6-ounce) grouper fillets
1 teaspoon olive oil

1 1/2 pounds asparagus
1 teaspoon olive oil
Salt and pepper

2 peaches, pitted and finely diced
1/4 cup onion, diced
2 tablespoon mint, chopped
Juice and zest of 1 lime
1/4 teaspoon salt
1 teaspoon olive oil

Heat your oven to 350 degrees F.

Place the fish on a plate and pat dry on both sides with paper towels. Season with salt and pepper on both sides.

Heat 1 teaspoon olive oil in a medium sauté pan over medium-high heat and sauté the fillets, two at a time, for 3 minutes on each side until golden brown. Remove to a baking sheet and repeat with the other 2 fillets. Bake the fish for 8 to 10 minutes, until done.

Toss the asparagus in a shallow baking pan with 1 teaspoon olive oil, salt and pepper, and roast for 8 to 10 minutes until tender.

In a mixing bowl, combine the peaches, onion, mint, the lime juice, zest, salt and olive oil, then cover and refrigerate until ready to serve.

Arrange the asparagus on a plate, then add the fish and top with a portion of the peach relish.

Grilled Grouper with Avocado Relish
and Snow Peas (4 servings)

Cals: 533   carbs: 15   sugar: 6   fat: 27   protein: 49

4 (6-ounce) grouper fillets

1 teaspoon olive oil
1 1/2 pounds snow peas
Salt and pepper

3 avocados, peeled, pitted and diced
1 tablespoon lime juice
1 tablespoon cilantro, chopped
1 tablespoon parsley, chopped
1 teaspoon olive oil
6 tablespoons red onion, diced
Salt and pepper to taste

Heat a grill to medium hot, 350 degrees F.

Season the grouper with salt and pepper on each side and grill 4 to 5 minutes on each side. Transfer the fish to a pan and cover with foil to keep warm until you are ready to serve.

Heat 1 teaspoon olive oil in a sauté pan over medium-high heat and cook the snow peas for 4 to 5 minutes, stirring frequently. Season with salt and pepper.

Stir together the avocados, lime juice, cilantro, parsley, olive oil, diced red onions, salt and pepper in a mixing bowl. .

Place the snow peas on a plate. Add the fi   and top with the avocado relish.

Baked Haddock with Broccoli Rabe
and Curried Lentils (4 servings)

Cals: 275 carbs: 13 sugar: 3 fat: 7 protein: 36

4 (6-ounce) haddock fillets
Salt and pepper

I pound broccoli rabe, trimmed
I teaspoon olive oil
Salt and pepper

I (12- to 16-ounce) can organic lentils
I tablespoon lemon juice
I teaspoon curry powder
I tablespoon cilantro, chopped
I teaspoon olive oil
Salt and pepper

Preheat your oven to 350 degrees F.

Season the haddock fillets on both sides with salt and pepper and bake in a shallow baking pan for 8 to 10 minutes until done.

Fill a large, deep-sided saucepan halfway with water, add the salt, and bring to a boil over high heat. Add the broccoli rabe and blanch for 3 minutes. Drain, and dry the rabe on paper towels.

Add the rabe and the olive oil to a sauté pan over medium-high heat and cook for 2 minutes to finish. Season with salt and pepper to taste.

Drain and rinse the lentils and add to a medium mixing bowl with the lime juice, curry, cilantro, olive oil, salt and pepper.

Place the broccoli rabe and the fish on a plate and top with the lentil mixture.

Baked Flounder with Bok Choy
and Sesame Tomato Relish (4 servings)

Cals: 249 carbs: 6 sugar: 2 fat: 10 protein: 33

4 (6-ounce) flounder fillets
Salt and pepper
1 teaspoon lemon juice

1 teaspoon olive oil
1 teaspoon garlic, chopped
1 1/2 pounds baby bok choy, trimmed and chopped in 1-inch pieces
Salt and pepper

1/2 pint cherry tomatoes, halved
2 teaspoon lemon juice
1 teaspoon sesame oil
1 teaspoon black sesame seeds
1 tablespoon basil, chopped
Salt and pepper to taste

Preheat your oven to 350 degrees F.

In a baking pan, season the fish fillets on both sides with salt and pepper. Pour the lemon juice over the fish and bake for 8 to 10 minutes, or until done.

Heat the olive oil in a sauté pan over medium-high heat and cook the garlic for 30 seconds. Add the bok choy and cook for 5 minutes, stirring frequently. Season with salt and pepper and set aside.

In a small bowl, mix together the sliced cherry tomatoes, lemon juice, sesame oil, sesame seeds, basil, salt and pepper.

Place a bed of bok choy on the plate. Put the flounder on top, and cover with sesame tomato relish.

Beef Tenderloin with Shiitake Mushrooms and Grilled Asparagus (4 servings)

Cals: 443   carbs: 11   sugar: 2   fat: 27   protein: 39

4 (6-ounce) beef tenderloins
Kosher salt
Pepper to taste
1 teaspoon fresh thyme, chopped
1 ½ pounds asparagus, trimmed
½ pound shiitake mushrooms, sliced
1 tablespoon olive oil

Season the beef with salt, pepper and thyme, and let stand at room temperature for 20 minutes.

Heat your grill to 400 degrees F and heat your oven to 400 degrees F.

Roast the asparagus in a shallow pan for 8 to 10 minutes.

Grill the tenderloins for 7 minutes, then turn and grill the other side 4 to 5 minutes for medium rare. Let the tenderloins rest for 8 to 10 minutes before slicing or serving.

To make the mushrooms, heat the olive oil in a sauté pan on medium-high heat. Add the mushrooms and sauté 5 to 7 minutes, stirring frequently.

Black Bean Relish (4 servings)

Cals: 118   carbs: 21   sugar: 2   fat: 2   protein: 7

1 (15-ounce) can black beans
1 tablespoon red onion, diced
1 teaspoon pureed garlic (see p. 164 for recipe)
1 tablespoon cilantro leaves, chopped
1 teaspoon olive oil
Salt and pepper to taste

Drain the beans and rinse with water. Combine all ingredients, mix thoroughly, and serve.

Braised Chicken Thighs with Fennel, Tomato and White Asparagus (4 servings)

Cals: 419   carbs: 23   sugar: 9   fat: 14   protein: 51

8 chicken thighs
Salt and pepper to taste
1 teaspoon olive oil
1 fennel bulb, thinly sliced
1 tablespoon pureed garlic (see p. 164 for recipe)
2 (15-ounce) cans crushed tomatoes, plus the juice from one can
2 cups chicken broth
1 tablespoon parsley leaves, chopped
1 pound asparagus

Heat your oven to 350 degrees F.

Season the chicken on both sides with salt and pepper. Heat the olive oil in a large sauté pan over medium-high heat and brown the chicken for 4 minutes on each side.

Transfer the chicken to a small roasting pan.

Using the same sauté pan, add the fennel slices and cook over medium-high heat for 3 minutes. Add the garlic and cook for 1 additional minute. Add the tomatoes and broth and cook for 2 to 3 minutes to reduce the liquid.

Pour the tomato mixture over the chicken and bake for 15 to 20 minutes. Garnish with parsley.

Cook the asparagus in a sauté pan over medium heat for 5 to 6 minutes, or until tender.

Broccoli Rabe Rapini (4 Servings)

Cals: 31 carbs: 1 sugar: 0 fat: 3 protein: 1

2 bunches broccoli rabe
I teaspoon oil
I teaspoon pureed garlic (see p. 164 for recipe)

Fill a large stockpot halfway with water, bring to a boil over high heat, and blanch the broccoli rabe for 3 minutes. Use a slotted spoon to remove the rabe from the pot and drain on paper towels.

Heat the oil in a large sauté pan on high heat, add the broccoli, and toss to coat with oil. Add the garlic puree and cook for 3 minutes, stirring.

Brown Rice Penne with Shrimp & Veggies (4 servings)

Cals: 299 carbs: 27 sugar: 4 fat: 7 protein: 31

I pound brown rice pasta
3 teaspoons olive oil
I pound (26-30 count) peeled shrimp
I pound yellow squash, ½-inch dice
1/4 pound whole cherry tomatoes
1/4 pound julienned snow peas
I tablespoon pureed garlic (see p. 164 for recipe)

Cook the pasta according to package directions, but stop cooking 2 minutes before it is done, and drain.

Heat 1 teaspoon olive oil in a large skillet over medium-high heat, then add the shrimp. Season with salt and pepper, and cook for 4 minutes. Remove the shrimp from the pan and set aside.

Add the squash to the pan, plus 1 teaspoon olive oil, and sauté for 4 minutes. Remove the squash from the pan and set aside.

Add the cherry tomatoes, snow peas, and garlic puree to the same pan, and sauté for 3 minutes. Return all ingredients to the pan, and stir together with the remaining 1 teaspoon olive oil. Season to taste and serve.

Cannellini Bean Relish (4 servings)

Cals: 75   carbs: 10   sugar: 1   fat: 3   protein: 4

1 (8-ounce) can cannellini beans, rinsed and drained
1 teaspoon diced red onion
1/4 teaspoon minced ginger
1/2 teaspoon chopped fresh basil
1/2 tablespoon olive oil
Salt and pepper to taste

Mix all the ingredients together in a medium bowl and refrigerate, covered, until ready to serve.

Crab Cakes (4 servings)

Cals: 172   carbs: 8   sugar: 2   fat: 15   protein: 3

1 pound lump crabmeat, picked for shells
1/4 cup finely diced celery
1/4 cup finely diced white onion
1 tablespoons, plus 3 teaspoons olive oil, divided
1 teaspoon pureed garlic (see p. 164 for recipe)
Salt and pepper to taste
1 egg, beaten
1 tablespoon lemon juice
2 tablespoons vegan mayo
1 teaspoon dried mustard
1/2 tablespoon fresh basil, diced
1/2 cup gluten-free bread crumbs

Spread the crabmeat on a sheet pan and remove any remaining shells, then transfer to a mixing bowl.

In a small skillet over medium-high heat, add 1 teaspoon olive oil and sauté the celery and onion for 4 minutes. Add the garlic puree, salt and pepper, and cook for more 2 minutes. Transfer the celery mixture to a mixing bowl and allow to cool for 20 minutes.

When the mixture has cooled, add the beaten egg, lemon juice, mayo, mustard, basil, salt, pepper and the bread crumbs to the bowl, and gently stir to combine.

Form the crab mixture into 8 cakes and heat 1 tablespoon olive oil in a nonstick skillet over medium-high heat. Sauté the crab cakes for 4 minutes on each side, or until golden brown.

Grilled Chicken with Butternut Squash and Brussels Sprouts (4 servings)

Cals: 357   carbs: 22   sugar: 5   fat: 14   protein: 34

4 (6-ounce) boneless chicken breasts
3 teaspoons olive oil
Salt and pepper to taste
Juice and zest of 1 orange
2 large butternut squash, halved
1 1/2 pounds Brussels sprouts

Lightly pound the chicken breasts to an even thickness. Transfer the breasts to a large bowl and add 1 teaspoon oil, salt, pepper, orange juice and zest. Cover the bowl and marinate in the refrigerator for 3 hours.

About an hour before you grill the chicken, preheat your oven to 400 degrees F.

Cut the squash in half lengthwise, brush each half with oil, season with salt and pepper, and roast for 25 to 30 minutes, or until tender. Remove from the oven and allow to cool. Once cool, scoop the meat of the squash into a bowl. Mash with salt and pepper to taste.

Trim the Brussels sprouts and toss with 1 teaspoon oil, salt and pepper in a medium-size bowl, then transfer to a shallow pan and roast for 30 to 35 minutes.

Heat the grill to 375 degrees F. Grill the chicken for 4 to 5 minutes on each side.

Roasted Rack of Lamb with Stir-Fried Green Beans
(4 servings)

Cals: 867   carbs: 11   sugar: 1   fat: 53   protein: 99

2 whole racks of lamb
Salt and pepper to taste
1 tablespoon rosemary, minced
1 pound Haricot vert or French green beans
1 tablespoon plus 1 teaspoon olive oil
1 teaspoon pureed garlic (see p. 164 for recipe)

Season the lamb generously with salt, pepper and rosemary. Let it stand at room temperature for 20 minutes.

Heat your oven to 350 degrees F.

In a large, deep pot or Dutch oven, heat 1 tablespoon oil over high heat, and sear the lamb on all sides for 3 to 4 minutes, or until golden brown.

Transfer the lamb to a roasting pan and roast for 15 to 20 minutes, or until the internal temperature reaches 125 degrees F, for medium rare. Remove from oven and allow the lamb to rest for 10 minutes. Carve between the rack bones.

Boil the green beans for 2 to 3 minutes, then drain.

Heat a large sauté pan over high heat, and add 1 teaspoon oil. Add the drained beans to the pan and mix thoroughly with the garlic puree.

Shrimp with Littleneck Clams, Andouille Sausage and Kale (4 servings)

Cals: 287   carbs: 14   sugar: 1   fat: 3   protein: 38

3 teaspoons olive oil
2 bunches kale, chopped
Salt and pepper to taste
1 pound (26-30 count) peeled shrimp
2 cups chicken stock
16 littleneck clams, cleaned and scrubbed
2 links andouille sausage, sliced

Heat 1 teaspoon olive oil in a large stockpot over high heat, and add the kale. Stir quickly to coat the kale, then season with salt and pepper. Add 1 ½ cups water to the pot, cover, and reduce the heat to medium-low. Cook for 20 minutes.

Season the shrimp with salt and pepper.

Add 1 teaspoon oil to a large, deep sauté pan on high heat, and cook the shrimp for 3 to 5 minutes. Remove the shrimp with a slotted spoon, then add the clams and 1 teaspoon oil to the same pan. Stir to coat thoroughly, then add 2 cups chicken stock. Cover, lower the heat to medium, and cook 4 to 5 minutes, or until the clams begin to open.

In a separate pan, sauté the sausage for 4 to 6 minutes, then add the sausage, kale and the shrimp to the clams. Stir and serve hot.

Tomato Mint Relish (4 servings)

Cals: 41   carbs: 7   sugar: 6   fat: 2   protein: 1

4 Roma tomatoes
1/2 tablespoon diced red onion
1/2 teaspoon sesame oil
10 mint leaves
Salt and pepper to taste

Combine all ingredients thoroughly and use immediately, or refrigerate, covered, until ready to use.

Roasted Garlic Puree

12 medium garlic cloves, peeled
1 teaspoon olive oil

Preheat your oven to 300 degrees F.

In a medium mixing bowl, toss the garlic with the oil. Wrap the garlic loosely in aluminum foil and roast for 20 to 25 minutes, until the garlic is soft and light brown. Let the garlic cool, and then puree in food processor until smooth.

Keep the puree in a lidded jar, refrigerated, for 1 week, or freeze in an air-tight container.

CHAPTER 14

Resource Guide

CONSULTATIONS WITH DR. KYRIN DUNSTON

Dr. Kyrin Dunston is located in Savannah, Georgia and offers a variety of online programs as well as one-on-one phone, Skype or in office consultations. Please visit her on the web for more information.

912.401.0449.
trulebalancemd.com
thebikinicode.com
themidlifediva.com

EDUCATIONAL RESOURCES

Age Management Medicine Group
Agemed.org

American Academy of Anti-Aging Medicine
A4m.com

American College for Advancement in Medicine
Acamnet.org

Institute of Functional Medicine
Functionalmedicine.org

Life Extension Foundation
Lef.org

MEDITATION TOOLS

Breathe to Beat the Blues by Amy Weintraub

The Relaxation Response by Herbert Benson, MD

Resting in Stillness by Rev. Paulette Pipe

NUTRITIONAL SUPPLEMENT COMPANIES

Designs for Health
designsforhealth.com

Metagenics
metagenics.com

Numedica
numedica.com

OrthoMolecular
orthomolecularproducts.com

True Balance MD
truebalancemd.com

Xymogen
xymogen.com

SUGGESTED READINGS

Functional Medicine

Bad Pharma: How Drug Companies Mislead Doctors and Harm Patients by Ben Goldacre

Big Pharma: Exposing the Global Healthcare Agenda by Jacky Law

The Cholesterol Hoax by Sherry A. Rogers
FDA: Failure, Deception, Abuse: The Story of an Out-of-Control Government Agency and What it Means for Your Health by Life Extension Magazine

What the Drug Companies Won't Tell You and Your Doctor Doesn't Know: The Alternative Treatments That May Change Your Life—and the Prescriptions That Could Harm You by Michael T. Murray, MD

Hormones

The 30-Day Natural Hormone Plan: Look and Feel Young Again-Without Synthetic HRT by Erika Schwartz, MD

Adrenal Fatigue, The 21st Century Stress Syndrome by Dr. James Wilson

Are Your Hormones Making You Sick? by Eldred B. Taylor, MD and Ava Bell-Taylor, MD

The Hormone Solution: Naturally Alleviate Symptoms of Hormone Imbalance from Adolescence Through Menopause by Erika Schwartz, MD

The Stress Connection by Eldred B. Taylor, MD and Ava Bell-Taylor, MD

Toxicity

Detoxify or Die by Sherry A. Rogers

Food Allergy Survival Guide: Surviving and Thriving with Food Allergies and Sensitivities by Vasanto Melina, Dina Aronson and Jo Stepaniak

Healing Digestion the Natural Way by D. Lindsey Berkson

The Ultimate Food Allergy Cookbook and Survival Guide by Nicolette M. Dumke

The Yeast Connection and Women's Health by William Crook, MD with Carolyn Dean, MD, ND and Elizabeth B. Crook

The Yeast Connection Cookbook by William Crook, MD and Marjorie Hurt Jones

Your Hidden Food Allergies Are Making You Fat by Rudy Rivera, MD and Roger Davis Deutsch

Mental, Emotional, Spiritual Balance and Creation

The Art of Extreme Self Care by Cheryl Richardson

Brave Thinking: The Art and Science of Dream Building by Mary Morrissey

Building Your Field of Dreams by Mary Morrissey

Creative Visualization: Use the Power of Your Imagination to Create What You Want in Your Life by Shakti Gawain

Molecules of Emotion: The Science Behind Mind-Body Medicine by Candace B. Pert

Take Time for Your Life by Cheryl Richardson

You Can Heal Your Life by Louise L. Hay

TESTING COMPANIES

Alcat
alcat.com

Doctors Data
doctorsdata.com

Genova Diagnostics
Gdx.net

Metametrix Lab
metametrix.com

ZRT Laboratory
Zrtlab.com

About the Author

L EADING BY EXAMPLE DR. KYRIN LOST A LIFE-changing 100 lbs. and is passionate about helping other Midlife Divas create health, bodies and lives that they love. Cracking the Bikini Code: 6 Secrets to Permanent Weight Loss Success, shares the keys to effortless weight loss, health and longevity that she has discovered, giving easy to follow details of how to lose 30 pounds in 6 weeks.

As a Board Certified OBGYN Dr. Dunston found treatments and outcomes for patients unsatisfactory in that they merely masked symptoms and failed to truly restore optimum health. In Functional Medicine she has found the solution that will heal us all: True health and well-being by addressing the underlying cause of disease and symptoms.

It is Dr. Dunston's mission to help people change their bodies, their health and their lives by giving them the knowledge, tools and support that they need to regain optimum health. In this book she details the steps to achieve successful weight loss naturally. Her virtual transformational program, the Bikini Code Virtual Boot Camp, helps people anywhere jump start their weight loss by addressing the underlying imbalances that cause weight gain and helps people lose 20-30 pounds in 6 weeks.

Dr. Dunston is a graduate of Jefferson Medical College and the American Academy of Anti-Aging Medicine's fellowship program in Anti-Aging, Regenerative and Functional Medicine. She is an expert in Functional Medicine, Weight Loss and Women's Health, has been featured in media and is a national speaker.

Acknowledgments

THE CREATION OF THIS BOOK WAS MADE POSSIBLE BY the contribution and support of many talented and dedicated individuals who believe in me and the concept of truly helping people with functional medicine.

A most heartfelt thank you to Dr. Eldred Taylor and T. Peter Strayhorn for their expert coaching, guidance, encouragement and support throughout this crucial transition in my life. I could not have done it without you.

I would like to thank my writer, Lauren Hunsberger, for her attentiveness and detail in getting my ideas coherently onto paper. You beautifully translated my original thoughts into the written word and maintained their intended clarity and personality.

Deep gratitude to Bryan Graves for his talent, expertise and generosity in formulating the delicious gourmet recipes for this program and for keeping me well fed and healthy each day.

Thank you to Janice Shay and Michelle Menner for their expertise in editing the text and scrutinizing the recipes so that they are easily followed and enjoyed by all. I am grateful for the input of Lilian Marshall, Rebecca Terrett, Rocquel Correcter, Jennifer Walts, Donna Krohn, Marguerite Cucquet, Arlene Meyer, Pam Sterling, Mary Morrissey, Mat Boggs, William Schroeder and Scott Fuller in the editorial and creative processes as well.

I am blessed with an excellent staff at True Balance MD that allows me the freedom to pursue extracurricular activities outside of direct patient care such as this book. Thank you to Amber Brinson, Tabatha Padgett, Angela Usher, Sara Mustard, Kendall Goco, Emma Lowe, Cynthia Swords, Dayna Barnett and Ruth Cruz for your devoted and expert support.

Thank you to my colleagues and friends Anna Cabeca, DO, Mehmet Oz, MD and Elissa Greene, NP.

Deep gratitude to my artistic team of Ben Marshall and Josh Branstetter for their excellent photography and cover design. Jessica of Dollface by Jules for her talent with makeup and Nancy Lucky and Boyd Holt for always-beautiful and camera-ready hair.

A huge thank you to all of my patients, whose health and stories have taught me more than any book ever could and without whom I would not have been able to create this work.

Enduring gratitude to my children, Julian and Chloe, whose love, support, eagerness and curiosity in life keep me on my toes and forever learning, growing and staying centered.

Finally, ultimate gratitude to the Divine from which all knowledge, insight, blessings and transformation originate and flow. May I stay forever connected to and inspired by the true nature and source of my being.

Index

A

acne xiii, 10, 18, 31, 32, 37
alcohol 18, 30, 51, 73, 75, 79, 84
American Academy of Anti-Aging Medicine xiv, 165
American College for Advancement in Medicine xiv, 165
andropause 10
anti-aging ix
antibiotics 7, 39, 40, 42
anxiety 9, 18, 19, 30, 31, 48, 50, 59, 83
apple cider vinegar 104, 112, 120, 124

B

bioelectrical impedance analysis (BIA) 71
bio-identical hormones 7, 13, 33
Blaylock, Russell xiv
blindness 11, 27
bloating 5, 9, 10, 35, 41, 42, 43, 51, 91
body mass index (BMI) 8, 72
bowel problems 18
Bragg's Amino Acids 115
Braverman, Eric xiv
Brownstein, David xiv

C

cholesterol 11, 50, 166
chronic constipation 9
chronic fatigue 9, 30
constipation 9, 18, 21, 28, 32, 35, 42, 50
cortisol 16, 25, 26, 27, 28, 29, 34, 37, 40, 46, 49, 53, 60, 61, 75, 82, 84, 85, 90

D

dark circles 18, 20, 21

decreased sex drive (Libido) 10, 18, 21, 30, 34

dementia 8, 27

deodorant 77

depression xiii, 9, 18, 30, 31, 48, 49, 50, 52, 61

detoxification 7, 13, 26, 37, 41, 66, 67, 68, 71, 72, 73, 75, 78, 85

DHEA (dehydroepiandrosterone) 16, 28, 29, 85

diabetes, Type 1 8, 11, 19, 27, 31, 34, 41, 43, 51, 59, 67

Dyspepsia (heart burn) 9

E

endometriosis 10, 30

estrogen 16, 28, 29, 33, 82

excess body fat 5, 12

F

fatigue x, xiii, 9, 10, 11, 16, 26, 28, 30, 37, 49, 50, 55, 82

fibroids 10

fibromyalgia 10

frequent Illness 10

functional medicine ix, xii, xiii, xiv, xv, 4, 7, 17, 19, 21, 22, 24, 28, 29, 36, 37, 38, 39, 40, 42, 47, 49, 52, 55, 56, 66, 67, 68, 71, 72, 81, 82, 83, 84, 90, 92, 169

G

GERD 18, 51

H

hair loss xiii, 28

hair, skin, and nail issues 10, 18

HCG Perfect Portions 104, 128, 130

headache 10, 18, 30, 42, 50, 91

heart attack 11

heart disease 8, 11, 27, 50, 67

high blood pressure x, xi, 5, 11, 50, 61

high cholesterol 11

hormone imbalance 13, 16, 24, 32, 33, 41, 55, 61, 81, 82, 95

I

J

K

L

M

N

P

R

restorative medicine   ix, xii
ringing in ears 18, 30

S

seasonal allergies 18, 41
sinus 10, 18, 36, 37, 41, 42, 51
sinusitis 18, 30, 41
Smith, Pamela   xiv
Standard American Diet   27, 38
stroke 11, 27
sugar cravings 18, 31, 51

T

testosterone   10, 16, 28, 29, 82
thinning and graying hair   10
thyroid xiii, 16, 24, 26, 28, 31, 49, 53, 76, 82, 90
thyroid Support 76
toothpaste 40, 76
True Balance MD xiv, 166, 169

W

weight gain 10, 11, 15, 18, 21, 24, 26, 27, 28-32, 35, 37, 41, 46, 48, 73

Y

yeast infection 10, 18, 51

34727676R00109

Made in the USA
San Bernardino, CA
05 June 2016